Weeds

*A Health Journey of Struggle,
Discovery, and Healing with the
Master Gardener*

Jeana Anderson

Weeds: A Health Journey of Struggle, Discovery, and Healing with the Master Gardener
Copyright © 2023 by Jeana Anderson

Published by Debarim Publishing, LLC
807 W. Broadway
Spiro, OK 74959
www.debarimpublishing.com

ISBN: 9798987929070
All rights reserved. No part of this publication may be reproduced, in any form or by any means, without prior written consent from Jeana Anderson.

All Scripture, unless otherwise indicated, is taken from the (NASB®) NEW AMERICAN STANDARD BIBLE®, Copyright © 1960, 1962, 1963, 1968, 1971, 1972, 1973, 1975, 1977, 1995 by the Lockman Foundation or the New American Standard Bible®, Copyright © 1960, 1971, 1977, 1995, 2020 by The Lockman Foundation. Used by permission. All rights reserved. (https://lockman.org)

Scripture quotations marked English Standard Version are from The ESV® Bible (The Holy Bible, English Standard Version®), copyright © 2001 by Crossway, a publishing ministry of Good News Publishers. Used by permission. All rights reserved.

Scripture quotations marked MSG are taken from The Message, copyright © 1993, 2002, 2018 by Eugene H. Peterson. Used by permission of NavPress. All rights reserved. Represented by Tyndale House Publishers.

Scripture quotations marked KJV are taken from the Holy Bible, King James Version (Public Domain).

Editor and Typesetter: Desert Rain Editing (desertrainediting.com)
Interior drawings: Angela Compton, Abigail Wood, and Jennifer Parker
Cover art: Jennifer Parker
Cover design: The Unique Book Cover (uniquebookcover.com)

The messages in this book were from You, Almighty Father.
I dedicate it back to You.

For Brian, my dedicated spousal unit, who survived the
insanity to enjoy the benefits of the healing.
Raaawwwrrrrr

Contents

Foreword	vii
Preface	xi
1. The Struggle Is Real	1
2. Garden Chaos	9
3. Diagnosis and Discovery	21
4. Definitions and Moments	29
5. Complete and Continuous	39
6. Choking and Hidden Weeds	49
7. Healing and Hope	61
8. If You Are Free and Clear	71
9. Final Thoughts	77
10. Tools from the Master Gardener Study Guide	85
Appendix	101
Notes	105
About the Author	109

Foreward

I met Jeana in the mid-1990's working at a small private elementary school. I immediately tagged the twenty-something strawberry blonde as a flower child—not because of any 1960's free-love hippie vibes, but more because she was so in tune with the holistic gifts the Father has made available through nature. Her bright-eyed wonder was infectious and her energy and zest for life never seemed to wane.

I feel certain she must have inwardly cringed as she heated up the kindergartners' lunches or saw me eat my *excuse-du-jour* that served as lunch each day. After getting the children situated, Jeana would pull out her perfectly portioned, compartmentalized whole foods and actually enjoy eating them!

As we got to know each other, I discovered that she had been raised to eat whole, natural foods and to use herbs and other components in nature to promote healing and good health. This is all easy for her, I thought, because she grew up with these habits. Anyone could succeed at holistic living, if that was all they had ever known. I know now that I was making an excuse for my lack of discipline and education in that area.

How many of us couldn't stand having to wait for the day we would be out on our own, away from the rules and restrictions we experienced under our parents' roof? Out on her own, Jeana could have jumped on the candy wagon into a self-induced sugar coma. Instead, she chose to continue in the wisdom of her upbringing.

Jeana has a discipline regarding the health and welfare of her family that has expanded from her roots, but she has not been content to use only the tools learned in her youth. From herbal remedies to various therapies, including healing massage, Jeana has continued to grow and learn, in order to expand her means to help others live in better health.

With the advent of alpha-gal in her life, Jeana's instincts kicked into overdrive. You will see how invaluable the discipline of keeping health journals was to backtracking and finding the cause of her symptoms. And you will see how the Father guided her to the truths of her condition, in order to help her weed out other factors that were impeding her healing.

The book you are holding records the journey of this "flower child" as she followed the leading of the Master Gardener, discerning between the things in her life to be weeded and those to be cultivated. May you bloom and thrive too as a flower child in the Father's garden!

—Suzanne Smykla Osborn
January 2023

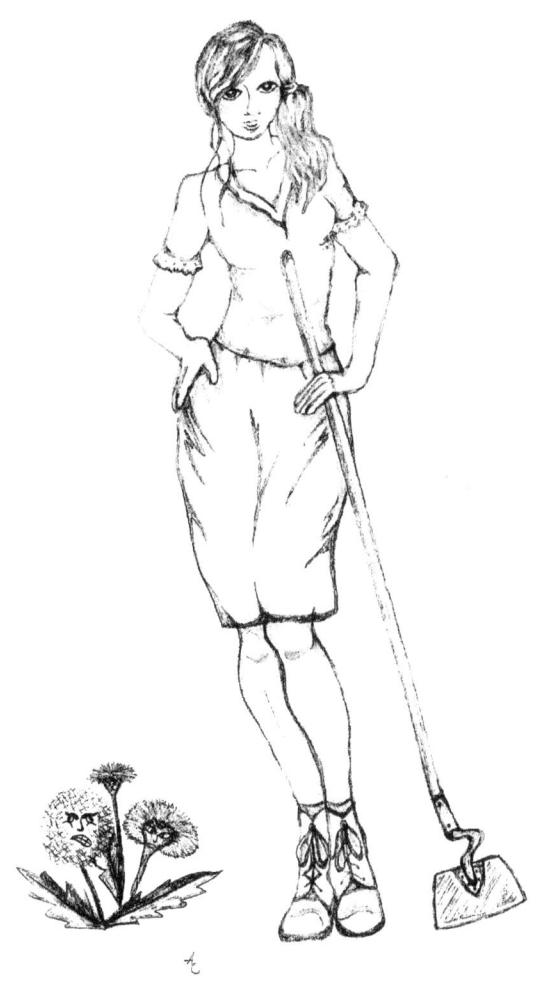

With hard labor you shall eat from it
All the days of your life.
Both thorns and thistles it shall grow for you;
Yet you shall eat the plants of the field.
(Genesis 3:17–18)

Preface

We want to treat symptoms, yet as they present themselves, there are deeper aspects to consider. We need not be afraid of the darkness; we carry light and the tools within us. Our heart of pain is the teacher and healer.

I have muddled through the past few years, filled with fear, guilt, pain, physical ups and downs, and mental chaos concerning my tick-borne manifestation and the varieties of sensitivities that came with it. I have found great strength and solitude in the midst of overcoming this allergy. I believe I did not see the entire answer all at once because my fears needed to be confronted first.

Fear would have caused me to go down the wrong path and create more weeds in my garden. I believe I have been given a path to walk with intermissions to pause and reflect upon each piece to this puzzle. And with each pause, fear decreased. It is okay not to know. Let the Master Gardener, who is Yahweh, the Almighty Father, guide you to discover the weeds only He can root out from your life.

Lives have weeds.
Lives have weed seeds.
What you and I need is a personal visit
with the Master Gardener and His garden tools.

Consider it all joy, my brethren,
when you encounter various trials,
knowing that the testing of your faith produces endurance.
And let endurance have its perfect result, so that you may be
perfect and complete, lacking in nothing.
But if any of you lacks wisdom, let him ask of God, who gives
to all generously and without reproach,
and it will be given to him.
(James 1:2–5)

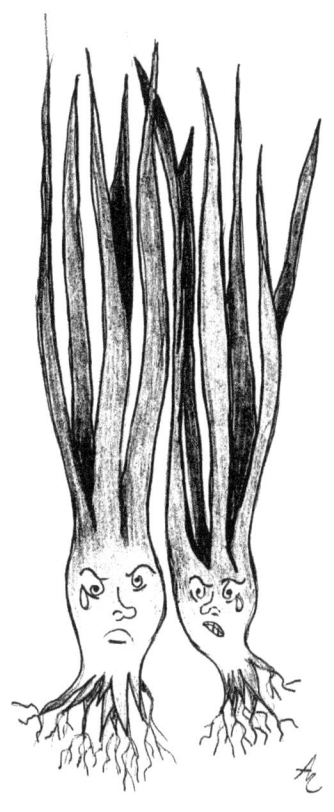

Do not be anxious about anything, but in everything by prayer and pleading with thanksgiving let your requests be made known to God.
(Philippians 4:6)

1

The Struggle Is Real

When you know that everything matters—that every move counts as much as any other—you will begin living a life of permanent purpose.
—Andy Andrews

My life changed so much seven years ago it makes my head spin. Overnight, 50 percent of my diet and the foods I loved were no longer something I could enjoy. I am not alone. My story is one among thousands. Alpha-gal rocked my world! It was mind-boggling! I have had perimenopausal food sensitivities, hormone food sensitivities, and more, but nothing like this obnoxious tick-borne food allergy. It is the "weed" that the Father used to inspire this book. "Weed" is the nickname I have given alpha-gal, and other obnoxious things that get into our bodies and lives. Alpha-gal syndrome (AGS), or alpha-gal (AG for short), is in its early research and did not even have a name until recently.[1] Some people have had it misdiagnosed for twenty to forty years. I have opinions and research on it linked to Lyme coinfections dating back long ago. Its roots cannot be traced easily because it slipped in unperceived, overlooked, and unrecognized. Like a weed.

Alpha-gal is carried to humans by ticks. Eating burgers, steaks, and other types of red meat will cause hives, swelling, and itching, or symptoms like vomiting or diarrhea four to six hours after consuming the stuff. The time it takes for the absorption of fat begins to explain the delay in symptoms.

On the surface of so many proteins, there are carbohydrate components of one kind or another and galactose is one of those. One of the fascinating things about this alpha-gal sugar is that it does not exist in humans. However, non-primate mammals—cows, sheep, pigs, dogs, deer—all have alpha-gal. As humans, we don't have that sugar, but we make an immune response to it.

When certain people are bitten by ticks or chiggers, the bite appears to set off a chain reaction in the body. The bite creates antibodies, and when a person eats mammalian meat, it triggers the release of histamine. Histamine is a compound found in the body that is the first responder to foreign substances; it is the cause of allergic symptoms. In addition to the classic symptoms, some people report significant gastrointestinal distress or gynecological symptoms, in the form of abdominal cramping and pain, heartburn, diarrhea, and nausea. Preexisting conditions can manifest to a greater degree than what they already were, like bone and joint conditions, adrenal fatigue, mineral deficiencies, menopausal issues, and existing food sensitivities.

The unrecognized dangers for those afflicted with alpha-gal are products like sweaters, soaps, and face creams. Medical products with an animal origin: pancreatic enzymes and thyroid supplements, magnesium stearate and stearic acid as inert fillers, vaccines grown in certain cell lines, gelatin, and some replacement heart valves grown in pigs.

Ranchers (who were unaware of their alpha-gal diagnosis) developed hives and swelling and had difficulty breathing after being splashed with amniotic fluid while they were helping calves to be born. Allergists have treated hunters who developed reactions after being covered with blood after field dressing deer; those cases raise the possibility that meat-processing workers could be at risk as well. School cafeteria workers have had reactions from breathing the fumes of meat cooking; the fumes are a common cause of AG symptoms. People with alpha-gal allergy may have greater allergic reactions to the stings of bees and wasps, potentially endangering landscapers and other outdoor workers.

I have personally experienced many of these situations and more. The bottom line is—once you get alpha-gal, eating meat from mammals and eating mammal products like milk, butter, yogurt, gelatin, etc., or using products with mammal components in them, can be minor to fatal. Alpha-gal alone is challenging, but when it creates an additional list of disorders, it can make simple, everyday life activities complex. You can read more about alpha-gal from the many resources in my appendix.

So, how has all this affected me you may ask? Stories are the best way to explain. On one occasion after my diagnosis, the family decided to go river kayaking. We arrived at the destination, and I got out the sunscreen. I remembered one big thing I needed to check—ingredients. Reading ingredients had become vital to my survival since my diagnosis of alpha-gal. I read the ingredients only to find the sunscreen had glycerin in it and found nowhere on the package the words "vegan," "vegetable-based products," or "vegetable glycerin." Glycerin is not always vegetable-based; if the product does not say, you do not know.

I had to decide: take the risk of an allergic reaction by using the product or cover up the best I could and take the risk of being sunburned. What would you do? I took the burn risk that day. I had a long-sleeved swim shirt and a huge garden hat, so I knew I had upper body protection, but I had nothing for my legs. After an hour on the water, I decided I needed to cover my legs. I remembered my towel in the dry bag, got it out and used it for the remaining hours we were on the water. I thought I might have avoided the burn, but each time I took the towel off my legs, they revealed the hour of sun had gotten the better of them. By the end of the day, I had exceptionally red thighs! It could have been worse if I had not covered well elsewhere. If I had not had a long-sleeved shirt, a big hat, and towel for cover, I would have chosen to stay behind and not gone on the river because the risk of using the sunscreen was greater. I purchased non-mammal sunscreens and skin products after that day.

The struggle is real, especially with food allergies. We must make decisions that alter little things and, sometimes, an entire plan. We must cook separate meals for ourselves, take "our" food and drinks everywhere, ask people to change their food choices while we are around, and the list goes on. Eating out is not easy with food issues. Let me give you two examples of food struggles I've encountered while eating out.

THE STRUGGLE IS REAL

The day I burned while kayaking, we had been on the water longer than expected and didn't get loaded up until 5 p.m. We decided to stop at Ruby Tuesday on our way home. I ordered the turkey burger with substitutions for the cheese and dairy dressing. I had to add the request that it be cooked on a safe grill (not being used to cook any mammal meats). To my surprise, they had recently trained the staff with a special "allergy" grill. Yes! You read that right. They have a special allergy grill and pans that are cleaned after each use and used only for food allergy requests. They had gluten-free/dairy-free/egg-free bread (wheat and egg allergy was a side effect of AG and Lyme affliction) that tasted great and held together. The fact that they had a plan for people like me already in place helped me to get through the struggle of it all. I name the place because they are taking many strides to make it easier for people with food allergies to enjoy eating out, as are many other places, and I hope to see many more do the same.

On another occasion, we were vacationing in Rochester, New York. It is difficult to know if a place will be safe until I walk in. I looked at the menu, saw the grills in the kitchen, and decided I needed to go back to the hotel and get "my food" while the rest of my family ate there. I was visibly disappointed. But before I could leave, the observant lady behind the counter said, "How can we make this work for you?" I was in the beginning stages of this issue, still upset about it all, and really did not want to trouble them. She insisted. I explained what my issue was, and she said they would create a new menu item and cook it in clean pans. I was emotional, humbled, and taken aback that they would go out of their way for my issue. It was amazing! It was a turning point for me in my attitude toward the allergy. I took on a new outlook on my issue and decided to take it on instead of wallowing in the negativity of it. Asking others to accommodate me became easier and more bearable after this experience. *Not* every place is like this. I have had some challenging situations that did not turn out as smoothly, yet overall, it has been a good outcome and a great learning experience for myself and others.

My mission is to help those with food and product sensitivities find positivity in what they can consume and use. If you (or someone you know) are plagued with AG, you are not alone. I will take this message to restaurants, activity coordinators, friends, and family members to be aware and provide options for these people. Life is tough when you cannot eat like you used to do. The more I talk about it, the more I find most people want to make something work for me. I have been humbled by my frustrations. I encourage those with no allergies to have patience with those who do. I know both sides now. The frustration and struggle are real on both sides of this issue. Shove the fears out and pull in internal strengths. The Creator of all does have our best interest, and He will make a way for us.

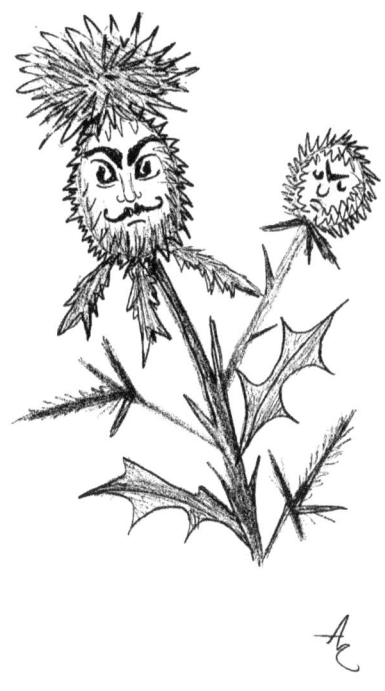

Blessed is a man who perseveres under trial; for once he has been approved, he will receive the crown of life which the Lord has promised to those who love Him.
(James 1:12)

2

Garden Chaos

Your minds may now be likened to a garden, which will, if neglected, yield only weeds and thistles; but, if cultivated, will produce the most beautiful flowers, and the most delicious fruits.
—Dorothea Dix

Gardens are chaotic. Sometimes, the chaos is in the eye of the beholder. It's either a mess or it's lovely. Or a combination of both, the same as with life. The trees, flowers, fruit, and water found in gardens provide us with both physical nutrition and emotional relief. The more diverse the ecosystem is, the more likely plants grow up healthier and more productive. Our connection to gardens is so important and is why we feel so good taking care of them. I was going through a turbulent and stressful time in my life and gardening became part of my healing process.

There is a healing energy that comes from bringing new life into this world.

I have written down nearly everything in both daily journals and health logs for most of my adult life. One of the best ways to see patterns and get a clearer picture of what is going on in the chaos of the body is to write it down every day. Writing it down takes the guesswork out, creates facts that cannot be denied, and helps others with information they need for investigation into a matter. My journal entries have captured unexpected twists and turns in my mind, body, and spirit I never imagined would have happened to me. Isn't that what we all say during trials?

June 2016 seemed to have been a time of much meditation. At the end of May, I had written about a load of busyness, stress, and excitement. I was transitioning from a part-time to full-time health and wellness practice, looking for a place for my practice, and learning about how to run a business. I was filled with anxiety and emotion from my husband, Brian's, long-distance travel his company had started doing more of that year. I had sleep and food issues I could not figure out. Struggle was my middle name; I had to push through each day. Memorial Day weekend, I was refreshed by two video sermons on Saturday, and my two teenage kids and I had a long video chat with Brian (because he would be gone another week). My kids really kept me from sinking into full depression by making me laugh and stay positive, while we tried to figure out what was suddenly going on with my body. Memorial Day, the kids and I played in an outdoor community band concert. We ate at a special burger place after the concert, and then returned home. I felt like I had eaten bad food. The kids had no reactions at all.

GARDEN CHAOS

The entire month had been a struggle with food and emotions. I could not pinpoint it to any one thing.

On June 6, I wrote a note in my journal about a tick bite on my right leg inside the thigh above the knee that I had treated for a few weeks. I had ups and downs with mind, body, and soul all that week. I had notes of the liquid and vegetarian foods I could eat and the natural things that were helping. I would get focused one day and out of touch with everything the next. My week was filled with teaching, volunteer classes at the pregnancy resource center (PRC), and trying to find a suitable building for my holistic health and massage business. I was overwhelmed and canceled an afternoon appointment, came home and took it all in. At the end of the week, I woke up with excitement because Brian was coming home, and I wanted to tell him about my vision for myself. Vision about building a business, coming to terms with his traveling job, and grasping the empty nest coming upon me while I kept doing all the things I love to do.

I felt good, but something was still bothering me. I did not know what. Brian returned late that night. We had one family day together and filled it to the brim with activity. Sunday Brian left again, and I knew what it felt like for those who feel utter loss and sadness when the significant other leaves for long trips. After eating well and having a great lunch (lamb pot pie), I hurled into a scary situation, an allergy-type reaction.

During the previous two weeks, I had recorded in my health log stomach issues in the very early mornings or very late nights, and that I was taking charcoal and probiotics to ease it. I wrote that I thought it was the tick bite from a few weeks before because I had issues every time I ate meat since then. Research of my symptoms led to some articles of strange allergies to meat after tick bites. I was not sure if this was the confirmed culprit.

Not eating suddenly gets one's attention! Instead of eating, I drank my food, and received some direction from an herbalist. I went on a bland food diet cleanse for the liver and small intestine. It was all I could hold down. I continued to teach my classes at the PRC, not feeling well. I thought maybe I had some mineral imbalances. Through the day, I had connections with people that gave me the same feedback I usually gave to others but had not asked myself, *What stress is in your life, Jeana?*

I never thought this intestinal trouble could be a depression thing but between my herbalist, Diana, my massage therapist, Shawna, a long-time licensed professional counselor friend, Kim, and the Almighty Father, I considered that there may be serious effects of holding in junk in my core. I prayed, cleansed, rested, researched, drank a lot of dandelion tea, took digestion enzymes pills, and listened. I had some realizations and good talks with Brian about my emotions concerning his job and travel, etc. I stayed on a bland diet, drank a lot of juice and water. I had a bodywork session and left with some new perspectives on my core-energy blockages. Was this all emotional? Was it the tick? I knew I must release the emotion to know what else was there. So, I came home, decided I needed professional help, and called Kim.

She listened to all my stuff and at the end of our conversation she said I was debating and refuting everything she said (I thought I was agreeing with her). She said I needed to digest her advice. I had to decide if my fears were true. Did

I have them after all? I realized I believed I had become "abandoned" inside, and I needed to know I was not abandoned. I needed to see and hear all the lies from the corrupt voice. My journal Scripture reads, "I have set my heart free" (Psalm 119:32). I had to do just that. I had to set my fears free: pent-up emotions against Brian, anger, hate, loneliness, abandonment. I had to truly give it to the Almighty, the Messiah's grace line, and find peace in it all. How? Why had I gotten this way over the past couple of years?

During this time, I was improving physically, sticking hard to the plan to cleanse and stay vegetarian. I prayed about what my professional friend said. I talked to Brian that night again about what I was learning. I slept very well! I woke with a less bloated stomach, a clearer head, but still not all on par. I felt sluggish mentally and physically. I realized I had been so out of it for days that I had neglected many important things. I meditated most of the morning; I was on my knees a lot. Lunchtime came, and I went into the kitchen to eat, make a salad with chicken and loads of veggies, sit down and took two bites. *Stop! What?!* I was eating a salad with chicken, food I had not eaten for days! I got up, went into the living room, got on my knees, and said, "OK, Father, I am not sure what has occurred, but I feel hungry for the first time in three days, as if nothing has occurred, and I feel I have had a physical change for good." I continued, "I am sorry for not giving thanks for my food. Please forgive me. Now what?" I looked out the window and saw the lilies, and said, "Oh Father, people long for what I have. I have not appreciated this place for a long while. This is my sanctuary; I have not thought of it that way in a long time. Please forgive me and put appreciation back into my heart."

It all came back. I felt home and loved it. I had hated being here for all the things I did not have (kids going to work and college during the days, and Brian gone a lot) and had been listening to lies that I was alone and abandoned from that other voice. I prayed again, "Father, please forgive me and give me a sense of belonging and inclusion." It was so. I had all the things most people dreamed of; I felt it in my heart again. Next in this kneeling moment, probably about thirty minutes total, was the most amazing part of the releases I needed: I said, "Fill me up. Crowd it out." I had many things come to mind including hate of Brian's job, business failures, body issues, just to name a few. Yet I said, "I must accept." I said those two things repeatedly. I said, "I will accept the way it is right now. I will live each moment. Fill me up. Crowd it out." I stood tall, faced every window, stood out in the light, breathed Him in, knelt back down and spoke. "Thank you." My stomach was flat again, my head clear as if nothing had occurred, and all symptoms of the past few days or weeks were gone.

I had been a complete and total captive of core emotional baggage over the years and did not even know it had occurred. Health is heart, mind, soul, body, and balance all together. I sat down to eat my beautiful salad and smiled. I messaged Diana. I messaged Kim. I had not even finished my lunch when Brian messaged me to ask if I wanted to go to New York with him for the week. I was amazed! His job was ending early, and he wanted me to fly there for a short vacation. My brain went frantic. I had wasted so much time being depressed that I had neglected important duties that were due that next week, and my classes at PRC were still going. I had a frantic time trying to figure out how to make a trip work. But I figured it out, got the garden prepped for my two weeks' absence, and got busy packing and planning. I had been in a depressive, non-productive state of being for weeks (maybe months or years), and within three days and two hours of giving my entire junk to the Father through the spirit, I was refreshed and awake as if nothing had been wrong. I had a new outlook.

That was not the end of the story in any way, shape, or form. Physical issues can be opened by life issues, fears, trauma, and vice versa. I wrote one day in July 2016:

Each page of my life seems to be a different life altogether. Each day seems to be as if I am beginning again; and, yet, it all seems to overlap and piece together at the same time.

After that week of awakening, my awareness had increased and stayed high. It is in these times of lift that we can have the biggest letdowns and hurtle downward faster than we came out. I still had food issues all year long, as my health logs show. I had to continuously deal with Brian's traveling job, and I had to keep moving forward when my business seemed to hit roadblocks. Renewal is a new level of thinking. Healing means I have to work to stay that way. Healing means physical ailments are gone, but they can resurface. From mid 2016 through August 2017, I had repeated phrases like, "great things occurring, made some connections." The falls and obstacles became important steps for my increasing awareness, direction, listening to my physical gut, and heightened spirituality. I have connected the gut to Almighty God. The gut is the voice, and the heart is the emotion. We guard the heart and listen to the gut. If I am questioning things in life, and feeling or being rejected, I put aside the questions and get back to the what of the moment. Rejection is from the heart of fear, and there is acceptance behind that fear. I wrote in September 2016:

> *I have issues with focus . . . I am so all over the place at home, and outside home, that all my goals are so many and none are completed or even started. Gardening has even been a disappointment; it has not produced for me, in one of the best seasons we have had in years because of me! How ironic. I have begun many things, allowed life to bring me down, put my focus aside or on other things, and the things that matter are in trouble or died and have filled with weeds from my lazy, lacking, slothfulness. This Is Not Me!*

How does that sound? Does this sound like the wonderful renewal back in June 2016? Well, let me tell you, the renewal took hold, and once all those releases were completed, another pattern was revealed. That is the way renewal works. It is constant and ever revealing. In fact, renewal is freedom so that more revealing can occur. Renewal peels the layers, kills the weeds, reveals the roots, and enjoys the fruit. Do I have worth and suffer at the same time? Yes! Do I make each day about worth, or do I wallow in the suffering so that by the end of the day I am not smiling?

From September 2016 to mid 2017, many people entered my life to lead me to understand my changing body and the recent issues it had acquired. My health logs reveal that I have had many imbalances over the past ten years, and many factors including auto trauma, adrenal crashes, mineral imbalances, and this recent allergy from the tick. Each thing added stress to the body. Things from childhood also popped up.

Month after month, day after day, I went back and forth with wallowing and feeling worthy. I had to continue to make the *worth* be more of the journey than the *wallow.* I had to clean my garden and take care of the renewal, each time better than before.

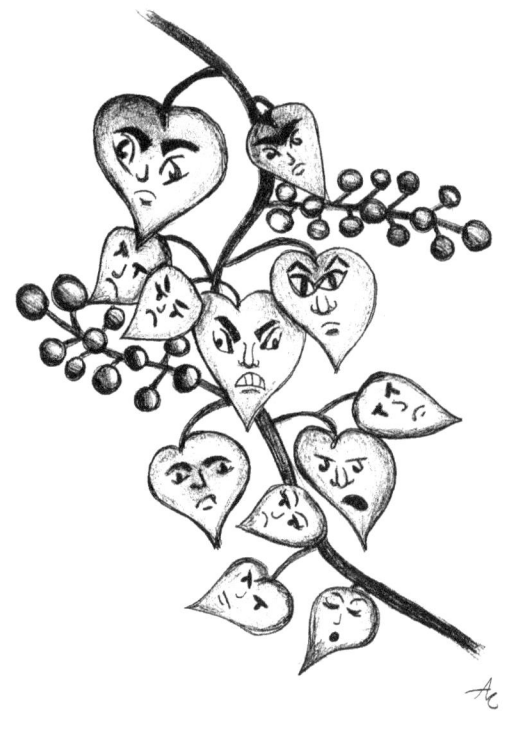

Come to Me, all who are weary and burdened, and I will give you rest. Take My yoke upon you and learn from Me, for I am gentle and humble in heart, and you will find rest for your souls. For My yoke is comfortable, and My burden is light.
(Matthew 11:28–30)

3

Diagnosis and Discovery

Learn the lesson that, if you are to do the work of a prophet, what you want is not a scepter, but a hoe. The prophet does not rise to reign, but to root out the weeds.
—Saint Bernard

On the night of February 9, 2017, I wrote: "Odd feeling after eating a hamburger." This is where my story takes on the biggest weed I have ever had to deal with in my life. Apparently, I had not come to terms with the fact that I had actual food sensitivity issues that popped up after May 2016. I blamed the body issues on life circumstances and was in denial that I could have physical health issues. I felt the reactions all over again with a sense of urgency: tight neck, gut issues, shoulder blade aches, and then they would be gone after about half an hour. I had eaten beef three nights in a row and I had not reacted until that night. I figured it was the bread, but I soon realized after looking back at logs that I had reactions similar after having beef meals more than once in a week. By March 9, I had been off beef for a month; I had been off dairy and cheese for three weeks. I had done very well with no sleep issues, stomach issues, or daytime eating issues.

But that night I ate steak and grilled vegetables, bread, and drank some red wine. After supper at 6 p.m. I felt anxious, so I took all the natural remedies that help me calm down during a reaction to try to be ahead of any reaction. By 9 p.m. I went to bed. I woke at 11:30 p.m. hot and sweaty, shaking, high pulse, stomach uneasy, and took all the stuff again. I was calm after the usual 30 minutes. (The funny part is I always had a bowel movement just before feeling better every time I had a reaction; Later, I discovered how common it is for people having a reaction to pass out during a bowel movement and realized my protection from the Father.)

I had brain fog for about a half a day after each reaction, which is common for people with reactive allergies to foods. By April 12, 2017, I had been doing well for a couple of weeks on a no beef, dairy, or gluten diet. I tried beef that day and had the same reaction as before. I also reacted to a meal with no mammal products (grilled chicken, green beans, and a salad), and this confused me.

With all the releasing of the emotional and physiological issues, I was not dealing with the physical issues of whatever was creating the chaos in my system. I took a food panel test (saliva and blood) to find out what was in me. In April, during Passover week, I received the results. I got confirmation that I had alpha-gal, a mammal allergy that included red meat and milk (specifically *casein,* a protein found in milk), as well as wheat, and egg white allergies. For a month or two, I tried to take out one food item and eat the rest, all with bad reactions. I reckoned with it and finally accepted that the diagnosis was true. In that time of wrestling with the reality of a life-altering allergy, I met many people with the same condition as me who never knew what they were dealing with. I have a strong spirit, placed there by the Father and a strong support system, friends and family, who were 100 percent sure I would come out of it. On May 8, 2017, I wrote:

> *I will not take a back seat to this crazy dis-ease . . . I will not live with it. I will not agree it is with me forever . . . I will not believe it is not curable. I will find the way to get rid of it . . . I have a characteristic about me that bombs an illness with everything in my capacity. I stick to a program until it is completed in healing. My daughter said to me, "Maybe God allowed you to have this so you can find the cure." I believed this, and I will put that thought into action as the Father gives me the path. I will not allow fear, lack of personal confidence, or lack of intimacy with the Creator to cause weeds to grow in my brain..*

By June 2017, I had figured out that even the cooking fumes of mammal meat affected me. I felt sick and had bad headaches after beef bacon had been cooked over the weekend a couple of times. I had to make rules for the house that there could be no cooking of any mammal while I was present. And any pans or cooking utensils had to be cleaned well, and the house aired out if mammal cooking was done while I was away. Cast-iron pans had to be stripped and seasoned with non-mammal fats so that I could eat what was cooked in them (cross-contamination, I later learned, was what caused the bad reaction to my grilled chicken meal). Transition to these new rules was not easy. If anyone made anything with butter or milk or meat that was mammal-based, the dishes used had to be cleaned well, the counter cleaned well, so that I could be safe in the kitchen. By July, I had to give up gluten as well. I was a vegan who could eat fish and bird, and gluten-free, egg-free foods. I discovered I had to use all-vegan personal products such as shampoo, toothpaste, massage cream, etc. I was discovering new things all the time that had mammal ingredients in them because I would have a reaction out of the blue. I had been on an herbal and nutritional protocol to clean out my body, blood and gut, and build it all back again. I had a big turnaround with greater management and faster recovery after episodes.

At the beginning of September 2017, I have a log of some reactions that were just strange. I had restless nights, muscle issues, brain fog, allergy symptoms, hormonal junk. I was lacking energy, snappy and grumpy. I had not eaten mammal products or used any that I knew of. Then, I read a social media post by someone describing my symptoms exactly and the culprit was **supplements.** Supplements can have magnesium stearate and stearic acid—fillers—which can come from mammal sources if not labeled otherwise. Also, lanolin in vitamin D comes from sheep, another mammal source. I had even been taking adrenal and glandular supplements (actual endocrine glands from mammals!). After stopping all these I felt better. I ordered all-vegan supplements after that.

I was stung on my ankle by a wasp in November. I had never reacted badly to stings before alpha-gal, but this created pain and swelling of my entire foot, hot and itchy. The swelling lasted for a couple of days before going down. That scared me. Having AG causes the body to go into histamine overload, called mast cell. It triggers cardiac issues; Postural Orthostatic Tachycardia Syndrome (POTS), where the autonomic nervous system isn't working properly; skin eruptions; joint pain; brain fog; and more. The less I triggered alpha-gal, reducing the other triggers, like histamine foods and egg whites, the more my body had a chance to heal.

Correct diagnosis for AG has been a long time coming, as you can see in the following excerpt from an article by Maryn McKenna titled "Why Are So Many People Getting a Meat Allergy?"

> In 1987, Dr. Sheryl van Nunen was confronted with a puzzle. She was the head of the allergy department at a regional hospital in the suburbs of Sydney, Australia, and had a reputation among her colleagues for sorting out mysterious episodes of anaphylaxis. This time, a man had been sent to see her who kept waking up in the middle of the night in the grip of some profound reaction.
>
> Van Nunen knew at once that this was out of the ordinary since most allergic reactions happen quickly after exposure instead of hours later. She

also knew that only a few allergens affect people after they have gone to bed. (Latex, for instance–someone sensitive to it might fall asleep and wake up in the midst of an allergy attack.) She checked the man for the obvious irritants and, when those tests came up negative, took a thorough look at his medical history and did a skin test for everything he had eaten and touched in the hours before bedtime. The only potential allergen that returned a positive result was meat. This was weird (and dismaying, in barbecue-loving Australia). But it was the only such case Van Nunen had ever seen. She coached the patient on how to avoid the meals that seemed to be triggering his reactions, put it down mentally to the unpredictability of the human immune system, and moved on.

Then a few more such patients came her way. There were six additional ones across the 1990s; by 2003, she had seen at least 70, all with the same problem, all apparently affected by meat they had eaten a few hours before. Groping for an explanation, she lengthened the list of questions she asked, quizzing the patients about whether they or their families had ever reacted to anything else: detergents, fabrics, plants in their gardens, insects on the plants.

"And invariably, these people would say to me: 'I haven't been bitten by a bee or a wasp, but I've had lots of tick bites,'" Van Nunen recalls.[2]

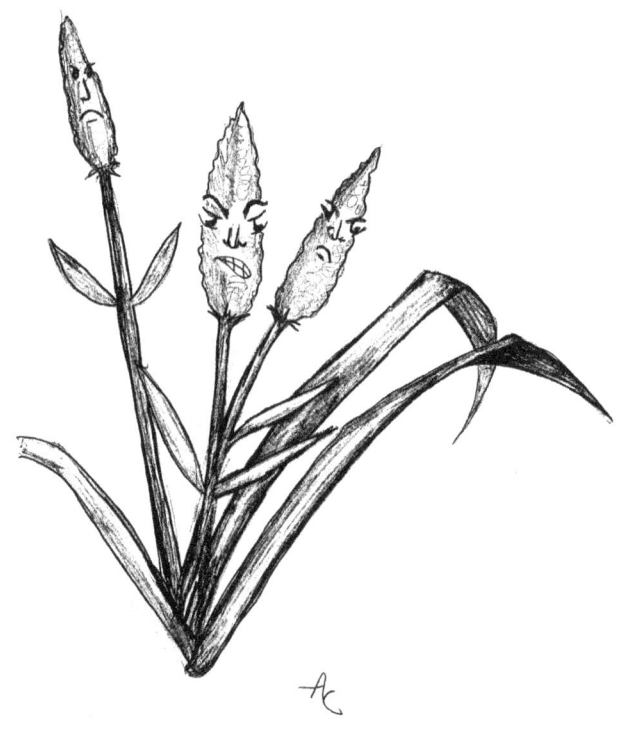

*There is no fear in love, but perfect love drives out fear,
because fear involves punishment, and the one who fears is
not perfected in love.*
(1 John 4:18)

4

Definitions and Moments

Is there anyone (or anything) right now that is a "weed" in your life instead of a flower? Are there any flowers that aren't getting enough of your time because it's being spent watering the weeds?
—Karla Davis

Moments define us. A defining moment is when you experience something that fundamentally changes you. These particular moments cause you to tap into your internal knowledge. Weeds must be dealt with *in the moment,* before they have a chance to utilize the nutrients.

Weeds are simply plants growing in the wrong place, where we do not want them or are not valued where they are growing. Weeds are commonly called invasive and problematic and have always existed in our world. Hosea 9:6 says, "Weeds will take over their treasures of silver; thorns will be in their tents."

WEEDS

Weeds can be found just about anywhere. While some weeds are well worth the trouble of removal, others are attractive and useful. Some wildflowers are nothing more than weeds, while others provide crucial sustenance to wildlife and environment.

There are two types of weeds—annuals and perennials. Annual weeds grow faster, typically spreading by seed and dying out within a year. Perennial weeds are more difficult to control as these weeds usually have extensive root systems that can cover large areas. They also come back every year.

Some weeds have rampant vines that smother, strangle, crush, and destroy everything around them. And some spread by runners, seeds, suckers, roots, plantlets, and bird droppings. Weeds reproduce incredibly fast; some can completely hide the surface of still water in a short amount of time. Many weed seeds stay viable, capable of sprouting after a long time spent in the soil. On crop plants, weeds can be partial or total parasites. Weeds harbor insects, pests, and diseases and compete for vegetation. They have the ability to grow in many types of climates and soils, imitate other plants, and take on different forms. Weeds survive damaging weather.

Think about the many kinds of weeds there are in relation to our life situations: certain aspects of family and children; unbroken ties to the past; assumptions, comparing, and taking one another for granted; ignoring boundaries, or not making boundaries; and our differing roles.

Many things in our lives that are accepted, natural, and look good are weeds. When preparing and planting a garden, the weeds must be dealt with. We, who are created in the image of the Master Gardener, can manage our life weeds by communication, sacrifice, creativity, and pushing fear away.

I believe fear was Job's weakness, his hedge. All he did, how he lived, and why he fell was because Satan was allowed into the hedge. Job lived "all right" out of fear. I have lived "all right" out of fear instead of being good for good's sake. This year's health experience has led to this understanding and forgiveness and truth about myself.

I am thankful that I kept a health log of my downtimes the past twenty years, no matter what it was, what I did to recover, and how I managed the ordeals. These entries are the end of the beginning to where I am now. Patterns and puzzle pieces were revealed through the pages of time written down just for this moment. On June 29, 2016, I wrote:

> *I have a pattern to lay out and learn from today, with pen, journal, meditative thought, and the Father. This morning in meditation and study I watched a video of a girl growing up dancing with heart but having mean hearts following her along the way (obstacles). She continues her dancing journey through it all, with a mother figure encouraging her, attaining her goal without resentment or bitterness taking over, keeping her passion in the dance. I think about just doing my thing without waiting on everyone to get on board. These things I need to pray and think on. I have never attained a goal because I allowed a stop sign to rule.*

I planned to find a way out of this tick-borne food allergy, alpha gal. I planned to help others on the same path. I intended all of this, but in the end, if all I did was put another piece of the path for the next to follow, then I would have accomplished much in the process.

My journals take on some patterns and similarities, loads of questions over the years, and a lot of learning experiences, which I have grown from. On August 6, 2017, I wrote in my health log:

> *Been doing much better when on a vegan-type diet (bird and fish meats included). Hard to do—miss dairy, etc. Sleeping and overall feeling better without mammal (dairy/meat), wheat, almonds, egg whites. I am feeling that I have had this tick-related food sensitivity issue for ten years, since 2007, when this health log began; I am not sure (and may never know).*

But my overall reactions in August 2017 were of being in a mental fog, having circulation and stomach issues, my head and jaw (or neck) in a TMJ (temporomandibular joint)-type state, not sleeping well, and having low energy. My health logs began with an allergic reaction and bite mark back in 2007, and all symptoms from then on are similar. After reading all my daily journal and health log notes, I found that in April 2008 I had a period of calm where all reactions and symptoms seemed to be in remission, popping up infrequently until 2015. Then, an increase of crashes and reactions occurred again. Maybe that initial bite in 2007 was a factor to all my adrenal and thyroid and intestinal issues. Stress was a factor too. Stress can cause allergies to resurface and functions of the body to break down. I believe blood type, stress, anxiety, and personal traumas cause us to be more susceptible to insects and plants and foods. Knowing this, I have had much greater control and faster recovery after each episode that occurred in 2017.

I have ups and downs in my daily journals and each one seems to match up with the health logs of reactions, with few exceptions. One thing I noticed is that reaction to food of any kind, and my emotional state of mind going crazy, seemed to fall near the fourteenth day of my menstrual cycle and then ease off. Then it would go into an emotional flurry the few days at the end of the cycle and into the beginning of it again. This very pattern in my journals was what kept me questioning for a year that I could have AG, or any allergy, before I took more concrete action (taking the food panel test I wrote about in the previous chapter). I only kept AG as a possibility because there were times of reaction on other spontaneous occasions. I also noticed that I had reactions after several meals in a row of mammal products, not just one meal alone; I noticed this gap closing as the year moved on.

I had to come to the reality that I had my first ever allergy—but this was more than just an allergy. I had the craziest allergy I have ever heard of in my life. I had to begin to process this diagnosis (in the same month as my forty-fifth birthday), declutter my mind, and receive the truth that was being revealed to me; only then would the solution become clear. I began researching and reading everything on AG. I personally contacted other researchers and people with AG. I decided I could not allow the allergy to become worse and began eliminating everything that could trigger it. For the next couple of months, anger, anxiety, and awareness filled my soul. I could not eat this, I could not use that product, I could not go into that restaurant, and I could not, could not, could not.

One day I was grocery shopping, a task I had begun to dislike because most of the things in the basket were things I could not eat any longer. I asked the Father for guidance to find safe foods for me, other than produce, without having to read every label in the store. I turned down an aisle—vegan candy! I had never seen it before. I turned down more aisles and found something in nearly every category, all dairy-free, gluten-free, and mammal-free. It was refreshing. On the way home, I meditated and chatted with the Father. I let go of the anger, depression, and exhaustive chaos in my mind. I turned over my newly acquired allergy as a challenge, and challenges are meant to be overcome.

Whether you feel like it or not, when we encounter a difficult challenge or *weed* in our lives, we must stop "in the moment" to deal with it before moving on. When I stop in the moment to take care of a situation, or approach a person with an issue, the result is always good. When I choose to not say or do something to immediately resolve a problem, it never ends well. Leaving the weed in place allows the issue to fester, strengthens the roots, and makes the solution more complex to fix.

Your actions can affect not only you, but also those you know (and those you may never meet). Ground yourself in the here and now. The body cannot be anywhere else. If we are not in the present moment, we are subject to false reality. Living life *in the moment* gives us purpose that the past and the future cannot provide.

In my garden, I work in the moment taking in every detail of the techniques I use: the types of weeds, the lay of the garden, the bugs, the birds, and the way everything merges. I notice my body's senses, movements, and abilities. In the moments of weeding, I make peace with the past, weed my mind of junk, smile, sing, all of which alters my attitude toward the allergy that seeded itself inside me. Yahweh, the Master Gardener, is there; wounds are healed, and I am present.

We prefer not to pull weeds, or deal with them in the moment, especially when it encompasses things we do not care to do. Weed pulling definitely draws us into the present moment, as does anything that is chore-like, yet it is necessary in order to grow fruit in our personal lives, and it is how the garden grows abundantly instead of being choked out. By attending to the moments, we have a better chance of staying alert and aware for longer periods of time, creating a purposeful day.

What do you do in the following situations?

- After a disagreement with a friend or spouse
- When you come across trash in a trail
- When you start to have a scratchy throat
- Or when you notice recurring, allergy-like symptoms

In the garden of life, whatever you water in the moment will grow. A message that came to me in the moment of gardening: weed before watering. Take time to check the garden before the rains come, or before turning on the sprinkler. Watering a weed creates more weeds, bigger weeds, and deeper weed roots. Weeds will consume the majority of the water and take away needed nutrients from useful plants.

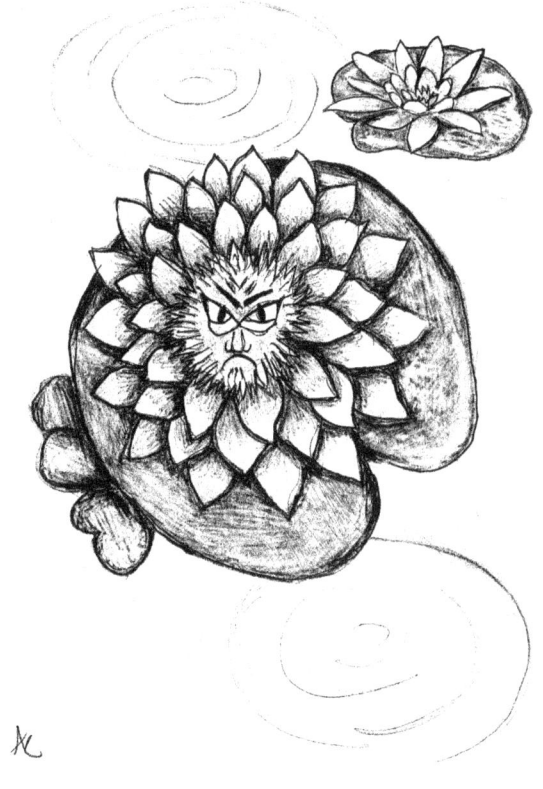

Let us hold fast the confession of our hope without wavering, for He who promised is faithful; and let us consider how to stimulate one another to love and good deeds.
(Hebrews 10:23–24)

5

Complete and Continuous

I've never really had any trouble coming up with ideas; they just grow, like weeds. The weeding is the hard part.
—Stuart Woods

When I compare my health logs with my daily journal, loads of patterns and realizations come out in both. In one entry I wrote, "slow down, be steady, and consistent."

In early 2017, my health logs showed improvements all around, physically and emotionally. In February I wrote, "I have had a strange few days, always an adventure for me during the week before my cycle begins again, things I have never had to deal with before but are a part of transition I guess." I further wrote, "Thank you, Yahweh. Please let me be a light today to all who need it, even if I am who needs it also." Positive business and marriage and family experiences fill the pages of February's daily journal. I find it interesting that I had all these improvements after making a clear move to be off all mammal products. My journal has some cleansing words at the end of April 2017:

> *Matthew 12 talks of a spirit being cleansed out of a house and leaving the house, then returning to find it cleansed; it brought seven other spirits more unclean than itself and the house becomes worse than it was before cleansing.*

This is how weeds grow. This shows how we must stay alert even after cleansing and renewal. Another journal entry later reads:

> *I am mending, growing, finding joy, releasing anger, and loving me. I am healing from the inside out . . . it feels great! Food changes, hormone therapy, massage therapy, new chiropractor, Bible therapy, eye therapy, life therapy is my life now, and it is fine.*

Slow down, be steady, and consistent. I had to recapture many times over the rest of that year and into the next. I am reminded of a time in the garden when I compared my manner of weeding with my husband's:

As I watched my husband help me weed the garden rows and around the plants, I wondered why it was taking him so long to do a row. I had done two rows already. I observed what he was doing but kept on doing what I was doing. A week later, we are in the garden again weeding. My husband was doing the same thing as before. I was finishing the weeding the next morning and it hit me: I have always done it this way, and he has always done it that way. I decided to compare the rows, and lo and behold, his were clean. I weed with the hoe and leave the weeds in the rows, upside down, or just uprooted. He weeds with the hoe and picks them up, puts them in a bucket, and throws them out of the garden. That is when the lightbulb came on in my brain. His rows are always less weedy the next time I go to weed. He is slow because he leaves little trace of any weeds. That morning, I slowed down and threw the weeds I pulled up away from the garden. I raked the rows of my messy weeding. I went down each of my rows to check for weeds I had missed. It was worth the time to do a better job. Weeding has been easier and less time-consuming ever since.

Weeding must be complete—the whole root and all parts with it. Get to know the rooting habits of your most common weeds. Pull the weed from its base or use a hoe to get the entire root. Make sure you root it up, knock the soil off, and throw it out of the garden. Weed the meager weeds, in addition to the sizable ones. You might think the small ones are too small to worry about. Some weeds may look innocent, but concealed beneath are the roots that make thorns and thistles. To get every weed out requires a lot of digging, pulling, and hoeing. Weeding takes time; it is worth it in the end.

Weeding must be continuous. We must be out in the garden daily to pick the fruit, yes, but also to take the time to weed. If we are weeding every day, then there is no chance there will ever be a takeover, and our fruit will last longer and be more abundant. Our fruit should rule the garden!

WEEDS

Weeding gives you a chance to study and make mental notes of what is going on with the life in your garden, to observe successes, to catch potential failures, to identify pests or beneficial insects, and to cultivate your best garden. Weeding gives you a reason to be in the garden.

Weeds in the garden are like the weeds in our bodies and our hearts; they spread out, across, and down deep. Weeding can be unwelcome, yet it must be done. When you weed thoroughly, and the area looks clear, there is a hidden seed in the soil, in the air, outside the fence, or in the corner somewhere that will show itself days later. It is a nuisance. And utterly downright maddening sometimes. Weeds can be managed in the garden and in life. It is not complicated. Good, loving management keeps weeds from hindering, challenging, or altering the face and growth of the fruit of our preferred vegetation.

Another cool thing that came from this year of renewal, after years of process, was a new outlook about food. Here is my journal entry from May 2017:

> *I have been in a restaurant with friends, with all the foods I love to eat around me; it was an emotional, crazy thing for me to order off the menu and creatively form a combination of food I could eat. I had a troop of support and help surrounding me and it all came out well! I learned at the same table there was another with the same issue. Ironic!*

I have had many episodes like this since, and they all have been easier to handle, and with a smile instead of a frown. On June 13, 2017, I wrote:

A year ago I had deep issues I did not understand, nor did I know what to do with. A year ago I had to let go of many strongholds and fears (body, marriage, grown kids, plans) and let the Father discipline, strengthen, and instruct! A year ago I had issues I thought were too much for me to bear, but weren't. Today, I am more free, more alive, and more clear with answers. Today, I still have holds and fears, but they are not permanent. Today, I can look back on the last year and realize it was not all for nothing, and though it was some wasted time, and though I got in my own way, I have purpose. Today, I am able to look back on ten years of junk and see the patterns I never saw so clearly before. In all of our expert professionalism, education, and experience, we never put together things we see now; the good patterns and the bad ones are all for the purpose of showing others, teaching others, and leading others. Today, I declare my purpose is to do the will of Him that leads me no matter what comes my way to sway me. Now, I have to act on what I have been given.

When life is going well, this is the time to be the most aware, and not let our guards down. Otherwise, we leave a hole in our hedge and weeds come through. I have to weed and tend my garden. I had to write all this down and give it to you. Romans 8:37 is the motivational power to drive our machinery! It says, " But in all these things we overwhelmingly conquer through Him who loved us." It is the life-giving power that shall cause the seeds buried within us to burst forth in the garden of the Messiah.

WEEDS

Weeds thrive in unbalanced soil and unbalanced territory. Some lawn and garden weeds bring nutrients and water up from deep in the soil and down from the air, and subsequently make them available to microbes and other plants. Some weeds break up compacted soil and control erosion. As weeds grow and die, they increase the organic matter of the soil. Weeds can be converted into something good for the garden community.

When I pull weeds, I turn them upside down and add them to the old mulch. They then become new mulch, good nutrition, cooling the ground for the roots of preferred vegetation. Many weeds, including their roots, are medicinal plants. The beautiful wildflowers that erupt around us from spring through fall bloom as otherwise ordinary weeds. Butterflies, bees, and caterpillars thrive because of these abundant plants. Some weeds have saved precious fertile earth from erosion, with little thanks from us. But toxic invaders (poison ivy), tough grass (Johnson grass), or perennials that spread by underground runners (sheep sorrel), you will want to root out. But allow the non-spreading annuals like spurge, purslane, lamb's-quarters, chickweed, and ragweed to anchor the bare ground. Good will come from it later when you pull them up and turn them into mulch or medicine and then plant your crops. Not long ago, top vegetable picks would have included lamb's-quarters, yellow dock, young dandelion leaves, purslane, chick-weed, land cress and sorrel; they have two or three times the nutritional value of spinach or Swiss chard. I remember a Mother Earth News article saying some weeds can work as trap crops, luring damaging insects away from valuable vegetables.

How can we apply this new perspective to life, with its ailments, tragedies, missions, and trials? Digest what you learn, make a plan to change, and act on what you find. You will figure it out because you are fearfully and wonderfully made.

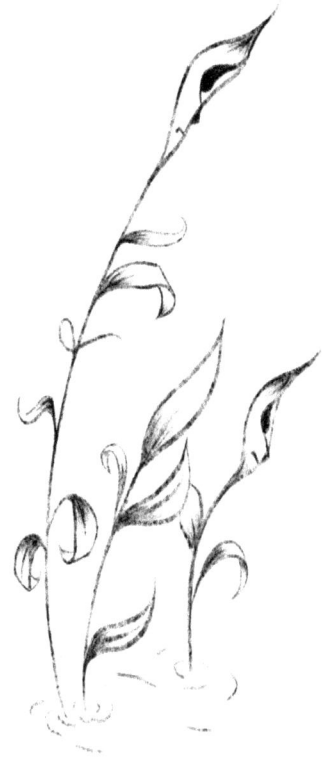

Others fell among the thorns, and the thorns came up and choked them out.
(Mathew 13:7)

6

Choking and Hidden Weeds

Avoiding action is also action, and its consequences are every bit as significant as acting with purpose.
—Andy Andrews

Weeds choke off the waterways and nutrients from beneficial plants, causing them to be prone to disease and insect infestation. I have trenches in my garden for the water to go out, so that my plants do not flood in big rains. Weeds grow in those trenches first because they are wet longer, but also because trenches are protection from the elements. These waterways must be weeded regularly or else the weeds will choke off the protection the waterway gives the garden. Weeds, even small ones, literally suck the water from the soil and the plants around them. Weeds will even stifle their own kind in competition for the territory.

WEEDS

After April cleansing and coming to embrace the reality of the plague inside me, and the renewal that was bigger, I became a mission-thriving human being. I wrote in my journal on May 8, 2017:

> *Praise! It is a new day. Brian has taken work close to home again and will no longer be traveling long distances and flying all over the country. I like this . . . Me and the alpha-gal mammal junk have met so many others living the reality of this issue this year. I do not take a back seat to this crazy whatever-it-may-be thing. I will not live with it! I will not agree that it is with me forever . . . I denied I had it, but I do, and I will find the way to get rid of it.*

I have a character trait about me that pushes and shoves if needed, and bombs an illness with all I have. I stick like glue to the program given me until I complete it and then I am better. I do not just "live with it." This world is in that mind frame of just live with it or tolerate it. I have allowed fear in the past to take me from becoming the teacher and advocate I have the potential to be. I was blind to this for a long time, and thought I was doing enough. I can do more.

I have had many say Yahweh, the Father, allowed this to happen to me, of all people, so I can find the cure and prevention, or at least be a lead for others to find it. I do not like this uncertain plague living in me, but it is what it is. I have had some great cleansing moments because of it.

Job had a gap in his hedge—fear was his weakness. All he did, how he lived, and why he fell was not from bad stuff, but because Satan found a way into the hedge; Job was a good man out of fear instead of just being good. Job became a teacher when fear was lifted. I have always lived parts of my life in fear—I have been good out of fear of rebuke instead of just being good for good's sake. The past few years I have been through fire and trauma to lead me to this understanding, forgiveness, and truth. I have a strong spirit in me, placed there by a loving Father, keeping me from destruction, and strengthening my senses. Thank you for using me this way, Father.

I have seen my good plants double in size after they have been well weeded. I have witnessed one good plant struggle and another flourish, only to find that the struggling one was cut off from the flowing water. In relation to my tick-borne affliction, I have struggled with mineral deficiencies and weakened lower intestines due to the massive reduction in what I could eat. Supplementation and herbal remedies had become a daily norm to retain my mineral and vitamin balance, and heal my gut. I was in a constant search for nutrient-rich alternatives to mammal products. Elimination of high histamine foods other than mammal, like wheat and peanuts, is part of the results of AG, but also part of the healing. I have dug new waterways, but the streams are much narrower.

I have a story from a fellow AG friend that can put this choking concept into more perspective. She had always been a meat eater growing up on a farm. She had many tick bites over the years and hadn't gotten bitten by a tick for a year before she exhibited any issues. She had anaphylaxis once and no one knew what it was from. She had another anaphylactic episode two weeks later, was resuscitated, and spent four days in the ICU in Boston with fifteen doctors poking and prodding her. They thought it was mastocytosis (a rare condition) and said she was probably dying from cancer. They released her to go home, but she needed six epinephrine injections on the flight and a rushed emergency to a known allergy doctor as soon as she got off the flight. There she was diagnosed correctly with AG. She experienced trauma from being misdiagnosed by doctors who just guessed at what she had on top of having a correct diagnosis that was just as traumatic. Her body has not been the same, her brain chemicals have not been the same, and she has fought against deep depression. She stopped dating because it was too embarrassing to explain that she couldn't touch them or kiss them goodnight if they had eaten a meal that she was allergic to. My AG friend quotes, "It [AG] can possibly be conquered, but it is a meticulous and careful pathway. I'm now getting better, but once you have the fear of death, you take baby steps."

I had been feeling fine with just eliminating mammal products from my body. I was a vegan who could eat fish and bird. Remember the wheat positive I mentioned on my food panel test? I had not taken that very seriously. I figured out the anger I experienced was stemming from the wheat I still ate. There was much evidence from the past ten years in my health logs that wheat may have been what weakened my gut making my system less able to kill off invaders that entered my body. I do not know for sure, because I ate only organic wheat my entire life. I eliminated wheat and felt doubly better. By the end of 2017 and into 2018, more food sensitivities developed. I had to stop eating all nuts and eggs. I had become sensitive to dogs, cats, candles in friends' homes, wine, and a variety of scents and scented products (not essential oils, to which I am thankful for).

I had a scary immediate reaction after eating olives at camp outreach in 2018 that included nausea, bloating, and cramping for about twenty minutes. After the ladies prayed over me fervently, I had a huge bowel movement and felt better; the culprit was lactic acid (a mammal product) in the olives, something most people don't ever think about. Going to the DMV and eye doctor in April and May 2018 revealed I would have to wear my glasses all the time, even driving. As with any Lyme-type issue like AG, it attaches to the pre-existing conditions and manifests them several times more than they originally are. I was able to read fine without glasses one month and the next not well at all, and I had to put that on my driver's license of all things! Sugar regulation and insulin obstacles had crept into the picture after June. There is not any solid reason for any of this except that the AG digs deep in the system like Lyme. I determined that this was not going to win, and I was not going to eliminate any more food from my already crazy diet. I asked the Almighty Father for an all-out war on this. I called in the Special Forces to weed my garden. I followed a massive action plan, the same plan I would follow if I had cancer, including antiparasitic and cleansing remedies.

Weeds can show up in surprising places: I am in my sunroom, putting new herbs into bigger pots, and adding new soil to old ones, harvesting some for drying, and preparing them for winter. I notice some of the plants look suspicious. They are potted plants, in potting soil, and yet, even then, weeds have grown. These plants were not transplanted from the outdoors, and they were not planted in outdoor soil. Thin, grass-like weeds had popped up in many of my pots, not many, but they were there. In a potted plant, you cannot just pull the weed like you can in the garden outside. In a potted plant, the weed and the plant have grown together, more than likely, and that is why I did not notice. The weed in a pot will have its roots intermingled with the plant. I had to cut the weed at the soil level and hope it would die off at the roots. I also have found weeds growing right through the rock floor I have in the greenhouse. The lesson here is that weed seeds are in the soil, in the air, and in the plant itself coming directly from the nursery. Weeds are part of a greater ecosystem. There is a Bible parable about weeds in Matthew 13:24–43. Thistles were found growing with the wheat. The servants asked if they should weed out the thistles. The master said, "No, if you weed the thistles, you'll pull up the wheat, too. Let them grow together until harvest time. Then I'll instruct the harvesters to pull up the thistles and tie them in bundles for the fire, then gather the wheat and put it in the barn" (The Message).

Alpha-gal, Lyme, and the hundreds of stealth microbes, have, as I stated in the beginning, come in from thin air. I do not know where, when, or how, but I and many researchers have plenty of guesses and theories. We cannot date this. We do not know if this may have been in the system of mammals for ages gone by that mankind was not sensitive to, or if it is a new kind of sensitivity that developed because of the corruption of the Earth and human food systems. It is a weed, however, that has developed like a plague, and its roots are in the ecosystem, intertwined with the mammals, encrypted into the human digestive system and blood by

CHOKING and HIDDEN WEEDS

way of a little tick or other species. There is always a vehicle, a medium, or channel for transferring one thing to another. "Weed" transmitters use these well.

Many challenging situations in our lives come in from seemingly nowhere. The reality is that they have always been there, and will always be there in this human existence. Weeds grow around the plants, but sometimes they come in from the sides and walkways. We can overlook many weeds when they are outside our "circle" of fruits and vegetables. Areas such as around fences where plants have finished producing for the season, areas where we have picked out the produce, and areas outside the fence. Weeds can vine in from far outside the garden, growing under the plant then choking it from the bottom up. This is where we have to follow the vine and dig the root from its outside source and not just cut the vine inside the fence. Weeds and grass will grow in the walkways and trenches, spreading toward the good plants slowly and gradually. We think we can leave them where they are because they are not near our good plants. But they rob the plants from that short distance and will eventually grow out of control creating a long, hard weeding process later, a too-overwhelming situation; and as a result, the good plants die slowly and fruit less. I believe the worst, most stealthy weeds are the weeds at the gate. Why? We put so much focus on keeping the weeds out, that we pass by the weeds that wait at the gate. These weeds are not trying to get in; they are attempting to block the way in.

The gate cannot open or close well with them there. Each time you pass through, the weeds and grass scrape your legs or latch upon your clothes. You have to walk on them, step over, step around them, or move them aside. If ignored too long, you are walking through tall, well-rooted overgrowth at the gate. The garden is not as inviting if the gate entrance is cluttered. The garden will be undervalued and the threat of damage underestimated with just a little thing as a neglected gate. Think about this in real-life situations. The list is endless and can vary from the places we shop, to our very own homes, from the things that waste time, to mental clutter, and from physical to spiritual health. We need to keep the gates clear physically, mentally, and spiritually.

Worse evils may be hidden under weeds. The weeds can seem okay where they are and not be a big problem. But they can be hiding some bad stuff underneath them. I pulled a bunch of weeds out one day, and it revealed a den of fire ants! I had to extinguish the fire ants before I could remove the weeds. We have to be aware of what is under the weeds. Snakes, wasps, grubs, and spiky weeds can be under or around a seemingly harmless weed. When there are groups of weeds, roots are deep, and they are tough to pull, but groups also create dangerous situations. Take care and be aware. Influence is more than interaction; our minds take in all aspects of every little detail around us, becoming part of our being, without us having any knowledge of it occurring. Fear, shame, negativity, disrespect, and an inability to engage in healthy conversation are some of the top influences that creep into our hearts and minds from seemingly harmless sources.

I have had issues that have come up in my life, but none like alpha-gal. In the process of weeding AG, I have uncovered many underlying things from my past that had migrated and blended into me before AG: hormone issues, genetic food allergen issues, and, of course, many things not even food-related.

CHOKING and HIDDEN WEEDS

I have adapted to, overlooked, ignored, and treated symptoms of these issues for so long that they have become "normal" in my outlook of body, mind, and soul. I am not saying AG is a good weed—it feeds off of the other layers and gives them more power in the body, and it is not the only weed. It revealed the layers. We must be self-aware enough to know we may be wrong, to accept our mistakes, and avoid making new ones. This will inspire others to follow our lead and force us to consider better solutions before we make decisions. In the midst of everyday surroundings, fundamental elements and essential people can be ignored.

Studies show that 70 percent of all people will experience imposter syndrome at some time in their lives. Coping with these feelings of self-doubt, we must try to find the right balance between operating with overconfidence and operating with humility. This is especially true with an affliction that affects your life and the lives of everyone you come in contact with. Fear and doubt are triggers that strike deep.

In May 2018, I wrote in my journal:

> *Garden is good, lots of good food coming from it. I am weeding, picking and eating out of it. My daughter and I trimmed the roadways, trail, and driveway. Fun to do it with her and use power tools. At some point that afternoon, after cleaning up, I found a tick, pulled it off, discovered three bite marks where the tick was. I had a small reaction that evening, but it was not the tick. It was fear and anxiety. It is scary just how these things can change a person's life (where there was no fear before).*

WEEDS

I have many more entries about this, even up to the present. I have triggers from past accidents, family situations, and life in general. I don't live in them, but they do pop up every now and then and remind me that I am human and that they are there. Yet, the Father is bigger than these triggers, and I can wash them away with the cleansing water of the spirit, just like in my garden.

Picture this: you are walking into a vegetable garden. You are enjoying the goodness of it. You have worked hard in it, sweated in it, toiled over it, weeded it, and cared for it. Goodness is everywhere, but then your eye catches something. A plant with loads of good fruit is nearly smashing the plant beside it. The plant with loads of fruit is so full that some of its fruit is rotting. Good fruit and good plants can become like weeds if allowed to get out of control. Get rid of the rotten fruit and stems, cut back the plant, and redirect its stems and vines so that its fruit can be good again, and the plants beside it can flourish. We must be detectives to find the treasures that lie in unexpected or common places.

I understand my life is a continuous work in progress; each trial, situation, or ailment brings with it greater insight and opportunity for transformation. How does walking in the garden scenario sound to you in relation to your life? Do you have fears causing your health or gifts to be smothered? Is there someone smothering your gifts?

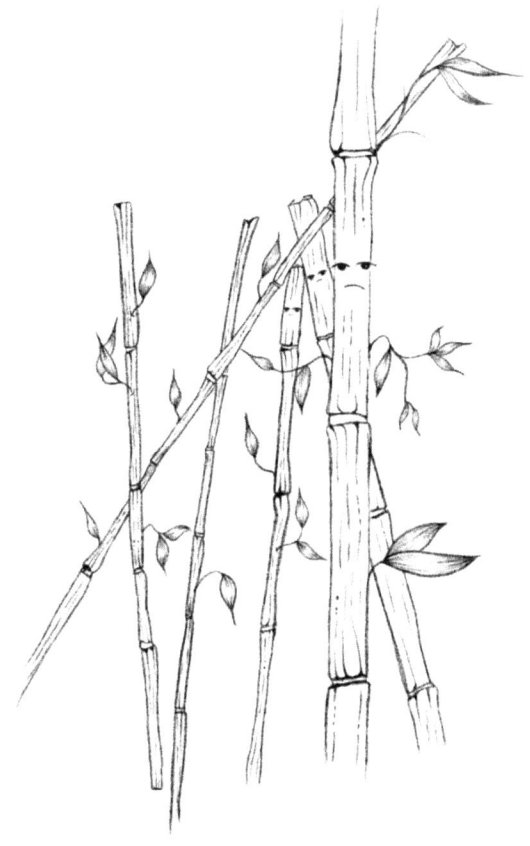

*Blessed be the God and Father of our Lord Jesus Christ, the
Father of mercies and God of all comfort,
who comforts us in all our affliction so that we will be able to
comfort those who are in any affliction with the comfort with
which we ourselves are comforted by God.
(2 Corinthians 1:3–4)*

7

Healing and Hope

An accountability partner is able to perceive what you can't see when blind spots and weaknesses block your vision. Such a person serves a tool in God's hand to promote spiritual growth, and he or she watches out for your best interest.
—Charles Stanley

I always want to be on the mountaintop, but someone once reminded me that the mountaintops are rocky and have no growth. The view is great, but what will it *do* for me? A view gives us a glimpse of the next destination. The view can stir our souls and give us a thirst for adventure, but to hit that target, we must come off the mountain, go through the valley, and begin to climb the next slope. It is in the valley that we plow through nature's garden—with its abundant vegetation and rich soil—planting, weeding, cultivating, and becoming what enables us to reach life's next mountain top.

Overall, I have had good things happen in the valley, and I can say Hallelujah to the past seven years. An encouraging and empowering outlook is what overcomes those struggles. I have always been healthy, strong, and spiritually stable, along with being downright tenacious and determined, which is why I believe I progressed through this recent trial with favorable success.

August 2018 was an amazing month for new beginnings on the healing path from AG, and other gut reactivity. I decided I was not going to live with AG, Lyme, or food and product sensitivities. I asked the Father for intervention and direction. I asked for the right people to be put into my path. I went to my chiropractor, Dr. Brown. He is not just an average chiropractor; he is led by the Father in what he does. We discussed my old physical injury issues and food sensitivities that seemed to be higher around the mid-cycle ovulation time frame of each month. He suggested that my repetitive physical issues had to be deeper. He gave me the name of Julie, the owner of a business that uses hyperbaric chambers. I drove directly there after my appointment, spoke with the ladies, and found my answers to the next step in my journey to rid this AG weed. Oxygen is key to ridding the body of unwanted parasites and Lyme. I had already been taking chlorophyll daily well before this day and eating high-oxygen foods. This referral from my chiropractor was Yahweh, the Master Gardener, telling me I was ready for the next part of the process. I signed up and began a forty-day regimen (five days a week for eight weeks) on August 8, 2018, eight weeks before Atonement/Yom Kippur (a day of fasting).

The timing was perfect. I had been reading about nutritional anemia being different from common anemia. Oxygen was the main factor in that difference.

Oxygen is the most basic and important substance in the human body.[3] Life without it cannot be sustained. Oxygen helps to eradicate viruses, bacteria, and other foreign bodies, and helps to maintain healthy histamine levels. The benefits of oxygen-rich blood include healthy digestive, immune, and nervous systems. We must keep oxygen in our bodies high. I had been having anemic and insulin-type reactions the entire time of my AG experience. Every person who is diagnosed with AG has similar reactions; however, each person will manifest their own enhanced preexisting conditions. I had to continue through my process of healing as my body's needs improved and changed. It was a meticulous, irritating process that lingered.

The thing I wanted most was to be free from the fear of food. Fear had a hold on my muscles, my digestion, my metabolism, and my blood. I did not want to fear my food any longer. My focus had changed from wanting to eat all the foods I had given up to a deeper one that asked: "Why did I want to eat them?" The ladies at the hyperbaric business knew that oxygen would awaken the body, clean out the toxins, and halt the growth of mycotoxins (a poisonous substance produced by a fungus and especially a mold) helping the cells heal and improve the immune system. But they loved what oxygen did for the mind of the person the most. It is a spiritual experience, not just a physical experience.

The time spent driving and the time spent in treatment was a sacrifice and a challenge for me. Yet, Hosea 6:3 states as early as the sun rises, He is there. He will come to us like the spring rains that water the earth. Each day, Yahweh provided me with new wisdom, clearer thoughts, inspired peace, and affirmed hope. During the 2-hour round trip and the hour in treatment, He gave me book after book to listen to.[4] These audiobooks were by people who had been where I had been in some shape or form of their own. They spoke to my heart, mind, and soul clearly, each one building onto the next. I also listened to Bible verses that focused on healing and living without negativity or fear. It was a great time of reflection and taking care of me.

I worked diligently on my mind more than anything else during this time. I knew that my thoughts, heart, and gut were all intertwined, and there had to be mental releasing and healing along with the physical. While I was doing my hyperbaric chamber treatments, I tried a 72-hour experiment to put my thoughts into place. Our bodies are influenced more by energy and the thoughts we have than they are by our DNA. I pray over my meals and those prayers put positive energy into the food, though I am not conscious of it. So, in my experiment I refrained from insulting talk about my body or AG or the symptoms. Before putting anything into my body, I prayed over it and asked the Creator to bless it. I infused my food with love, joy, peace, patience, kindness, goodness, faithfulness, gentleness, and self-control; these provide scaffolding for the physical body.

I had a detox eruption in the middle of the 72-hour experiment, along with several grieving events that took place in the same week: a friend's daughter had died in an auto accident while on a church youth trip, and a close friend and matriarch in our church congregation died. I had to skip a day in the hyperbaric chamber. I had to allow my body to grieve and detox and rest. My husband anointed me, asked to find what needed to be bound, and by the next day I was fine. My body fell into a calm with the deaths, and my mind was filled with the affirming words I had been practicing in the experiment. Yahweh, the Father, inspired this experiment at the exact moment I would need it. The results were astounding.

Bad habits were revealed to me during that week, such as eating quickly at the office or home, not leaving enough time to eat, and eating in the car a lot. After fixing that habit with time management, many things in my body and life stabilized. This was all within the first two weeks of hyperbaric treatments. Through the weeks of hyperbaric treatments, my ear and sinus cavities felt clearer, my spinal column and neck stronger, my shoulder injury was better than ever, and my thyroid became more functional. I could see the results of the Lyme and AG toxins decreasing because I was experiencing fewer reactive hits with less strength in them.

The last day of hyperbaric treatments, I made a promise to myself to change my perspective, keep my vision, and fear not. The next day (the day of Atonement) was a holy day of fasting, reflection, hope, healing, newness, restoration, and looking forward to all of that permanently with the Savior. When I broke fast in the evening, I made a plan to ease into adding things back slowly and methodically, keeping notes, and remembering my promise and the healing. I had to remember healing is a process. Healing can and does create an opening for another hidden weed to come to the surface. The two weeks following the fasting, my family and I were in Utah, and I asked for the entire congregation of friends and elders to surround me and anoint me for the completion of the healing process. I enjoyed trying cheeses (small amounts), and a few other dairy things, sitting by the grills unafraid of the fumes, feeling free of a crazy allergy that wanted to take me down, surrounded by the beauty of the mountain air.

After returning home, I had a series of reactions all through October that took me off guard. I was very upset and had thoughts that I had jumped too fast eating foods I had previously been sensitive to. I was having minor reactions regularly. We eventually figured out a mouse had made a nest deep in the intake of the air conditioning unit of my vehicle while we were away, died when I drove it again, and the toxins got to me. It could have happened to anyone. I am putting this little story in because the "weed master" does not want us to have healing. He wants to put that fear right back into us. He wants us to second guess everything. I moved through it and kept my mind from drifting. After the mouse incident was cleared up, I felt good for a while, and then spontaneous reactions would occur with no particular pattern. I would try something, have a minor reaction, recognize it was unconscious fear, and put it into place. I will admit I had herbs and oils ready to calm the internal reactions, and they did help, but I had to get to where I did not rely on them.

I am human, and there were a few short-lived relapses over the next couple of years that allowed the weeds to get through the gate. But I knew it was fear getting the best of me in times of high stress, virus, or perimenopausal hormone changes. Music helped me throughout the entire journey; my empowerment song was "Fear Is a Liar" by Zach Williams.[5] I kept the promise I made during that 72-hour experiment to "change my perspective, keep my vision, and fear not." I kept my focus as steady and thorough as I could. Does what you think affect your environment, specifically the food you take into your body or products you place on your body? Try a 72-hour experiment asking yourself this question every time you eat or drink. Write down the results. The patterns will amaze you and help you to heal.

In the beginning of my journey, I had questions/symptoms/unknowns related to food and product sensitivities. I made discoveries and had a diagnosis, and I found a healing path and a spiritual revelation. There is hope for the journey, empowerment to dig out from the weeds that strangle, and healing to be found. Yes, we want to treat our symptoms, but there is a wounded child in there, and it is presenting itself. We need not be afraid of the darkness; we carry light and the tools within us. Our heart of pain is the healing and the teacher. Meditation is mindfulness, listening, and this is a huge key to healing. I know this to be true.

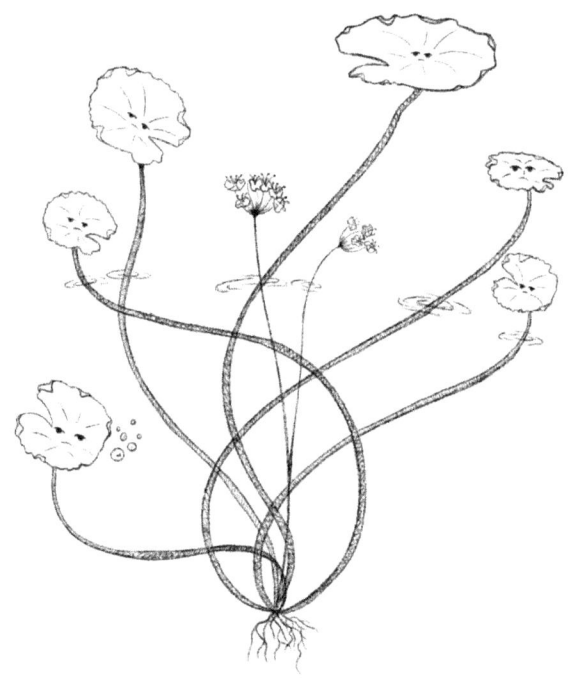

*So that there may be no division in the body, but that the
parts may have the same care for one another.
And if one part of the body suffers, all the parts suffer with it;
if a part is honored, all the parts rejoice with it.
(1 Corinthians 12:25–26)*

8

If You Are Free and Clear

Now might be a good time to look at your life and determine what's working, what and who bring you joy, as well as those that do not bring joy, and move in a direction that allows you to get the most out of your life so you won't become entangled by any weeds that exist.
—Karla Davis

The one with the tick-borne affliction or food sensitivity is not the only one having the emotional roller coaster or the struggle. My family had to stop cooking any mammal meat in the house. I had to mark certain pans mammal-free. Food products had to be separated and well sealed. When anyone cooked with mammal products, cleaning and care was a priority to avoid cross contamination. Household cleaning and personal care products were replaced with mammal-free products. The learning curve for everyone was not fun. I hated for them to go through all that. For them, it felt like they had the allergy too.

Helping people outside the family understand AG was even tougher at times. This learning curve can cause everyone involved to worry and to overthink every detail. People become worn out from the self-advocacy and constant vigilance that a food allergy requires. Whether you are the one affected, or you know someone who is, here are some important points to consider:

Prepare for an emotional roller-coaster. Tick-borne food and product issues can be life-threatening, so it's understandable when individuals (or their families) experience strong emotions such as fear, sadness, anger, or guilt connected to the diagnosis. These emotions can lead to becoming overwhelmed. Counselors say that equipping clients with coping tools will help them manage their own anxiety, negative emotions, and keep them from transferring those feelings to the child or family member with the issue.

Move toward acceptance. Help each other reach acceptance of the tick-borne diagnosis. Come to terms with the fact that you can't change the situation and take control of your story.

Consider your pets. Pets and farm animals are a huge emotional transition for everyone. This may be harder than food and products to walk through together. The person with AG will most likely not be able to be around cats, dogs, or mammalian farm animals. The household may have to give pets a new home, or turn half the home into a "mammal-free" area. Family members may have to take on chores of the one with AG. I encourage you to talk through these situations with friends and family outside your home as well, because there will be places the person with AG cannot safely be if there are pets in the house. With great care and love, you will find ways to make it all work for the best of everyone.

Explain the allergy. An individual with tick-borne allergies (or the parents of a child with them) will need to explain the allergy to everyone from school staff to well-meaning relatives who are hosting a family dinner. Be aware that there can be many levels of understanding and flexibility surrounding the issue. Parents may find themselves growing anxious as their child with the diagnosis ages, develops more independence, and spends more time away from home. But with a little encouragement, they can gradually give the child more freedom and responsibility to make safe choices independently.

Work with an allergist who knows AG well. A long-distance allergist who knows the issue well will be able to educate the allergists closer to you. Connect them. Many allergists have no knowledge of this issue. Many have heard of it but have not researched it. The more we enlighten allergists to understanding AG, the better. I personally helped to educate my local allergist, and he has become a great light for people with AG.

If you are not personally impacted by tick-borne afflictions or food sensitivities, why be aware of them in the first place?

Those who do not have food allergies can help by understanding the condition and doing their part to create a safe environment to prevent serious reactions in friends and family from occurring.

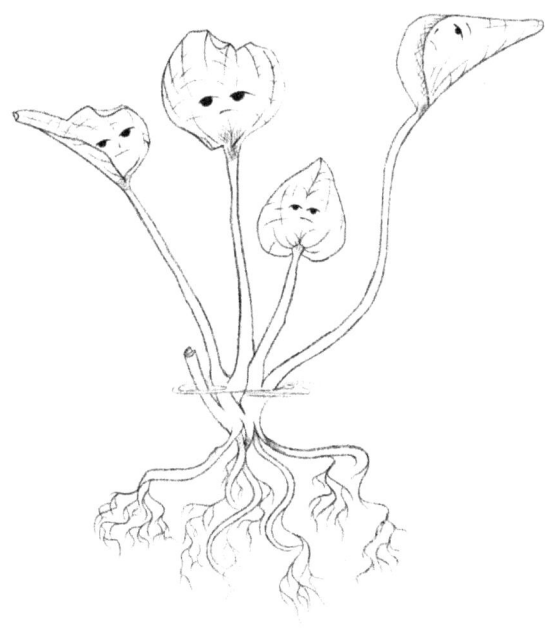

Finally, brothers and sisters, rejoice, mend your ways, be comforted, be like-minded, live in peace; and the God of love and peace will be with you.
(2 Corinthians 13:11)

9

Final Thoughts

Go often to the house of thy friend, for weeds choke the unused path.
—Ralph Waldo Emerson

Before putting anything into your body, pray over it and bless it. Infuse food with love, joy, and peace. I pray over and bless my plants also, and I see the results. I was the only one with a bountiful garden several times when the gardens around me were not faring well from the inconsistent weather. Prayers, productive thoughts, and mindfulness provide scaffolding for your physical body.

Accountability and Support

Weeding on your own can be productive, and depending upon your circumstances, thorough. Weeding with another person or a team, while still painstaking, takes much less time and can be much more complete with greater detail. Weeding, whether on your own or with help, should be performed with great care, with the goal of completeness; every detail needs to be regarded wholly, not superficially or partially.

Early on, when I noticed symptoms of something not quite right after eating certain foods, I began my self-evaluation. It was not until I began to talk to others that I became aware of what was going on in my body. I found a local ear, nose, and throat specialist and allergist for testing and, after receiving results, began a search for others with alpha-gal. (I found out that many of my friends whom I had known for a long time had the same thing.) I also found a support group. Support groups were my key to unlocking the confusion by hearing and reading firsthand accounts and finding solutions for the many issues tied to AG. I became empowered by the support. I connected with allergists who had more knowledge of AG, and gained insight into how to keep alpha-gal from bringing me down or becoming worse. I read everything on the support group posts and files, and I posted everything I was learning and reading.

I believe together we become stronger instead of weaker. Together we find ways to rid this weed from us, or at the least, keep it from becoming worse. Together we pray and encourage each other.

Words of Wisdom

Shame and fear are the bottom-line causes for all negative issues. They grapple with our hearts and minds. They attack our thresholds and tear down our ability to let go. We build expectations into everything. Expectations are not healthy no matter how much we twist the truth of the word. They lead to distress in body, mind, and soul. Expectations lead to unforgiveness with others, self, and situations that occur.

Unforgiveness leads to stress and anxiety on all levels. Unforgiveness is poison. The way to release stress and anxiety is to get rid of the toxins creating it, one at a time, pulling them out like weeds in a garden. Forgiveness, releasing stress, and serving others heals the heart (quite literally) and gives you your health back. Colossians 3:13 reads, "bearing with one another, and forgiving each other, whoever has a complaint against anyone; just as the Lord forgave you, so also should you." As the old hymn says, "Nothing between my soul and the Savior, / So that His blessed face may be seen; / Nothing preventing the least of His favor: / Keep the way clear! Let nothing between."[6]

I made a commitment to be in my physical garden every day. I have learned to see more fruit than weeds. When this is applied to the body, mind, and soul stress and anxiety decrease greatly. I recommend you pull one internal weed a day. When stress and anxiety decrease, the body heals from the inside out, heals the organs, heals the brain, heals the nerves, and heals the bones. You see where I am going with this? Joy is not happiness. Happiness is circumstantial. Joy is lasting, constant, settled, and not affected by the "outside" distractions. We have to roll up our sleeves, join the adventure, and take care of our garden.

I would like to add a small side perspective here, even though it seems a little out of place with the message in this section. When you space plants close together, it chokes out emerging weeds by shading the soil between plants. I know this is true because under the huge squash and tomato plants, corn in the field, or trees in the orchard, there are few weeds. Mulching is an important part of gardening because it reverses the soil tables of the weeds. Turning the tables on who is choking whom is a real "aha moment" in the garden, and in life.

Weeds grow naturally without planting or cultivation. Your mind is ready to grow whatever is in it. The writer of Ephesians talked of "every wind of doctrine" because he knew the ways of the weeds and how they would blow on the wind from one clean field to another.

We tend to avoid and resist suffering at all costs. We demand to bring our expectations to reality through various means. However, there is redemption and value in pain, illness, or any experience that isn't what we have envisioned for ourselves. Escaping from discomfort, or helping others do so, will never be successful. All of us are frail, breakable, going about life's journey. Think of the most difficult situation you are in right now. Think of that as the wrapping paper. Look beyond the paper—unwrap. Be thankful, unwrap, and put your eyes on the Messiah who was wrapped in newborn flesh and then ripped it open on the stake. We may not like the wrapping paper at the time, but think of the curtain being torn from top to bottom that separated the people from the Father and is now wide open, unwrapped (Matthew 27:51).

A wise friend gave a Bible study once. He said there are seven places in the first five books of the Bible where there is a command to eat unleavened bread and only one place where it commands to remove it. Seven commands to ingest the one Messiah who is sinless, and one command to remove sin (ingesting the Messiah is a metaphor for *believing in* and *abiding in* Him). The focus of the study is on taking in Him

FINAL THOUGHTS

who saves and has the solution. Remove something bad and replace it with good (or seven times good). Our nature is of flesh and spirit. The spirit should be seven times the flesh. Joshua 1:7 is a command to be strong and courageous, and Luke 12:22–34 tells us to look at the birds and consider the lilies—stop, look, act—and not worry.

On another occasion, I heard a sermon on the subject of thinking, reasoning, choosing, and believing, all of which we are created to do. We can allow the words of the Almighty Father to overwhelm us, or we can cling to the Author and see the simplicity. Challenge all thinking, prove all things—according to the Messiah's thinking—and all shame and fear will be put under His feet.

I have come to believe transition space is the only place that true change occurs; that space between one point and another, where we release the emotional holds and surrender, like a tree in winter lets go to make way for the next leaf or flower. Surrender means active alignment, not idleness. With all the fear and unknowns that can accompany transitions, they are still the most dynamic, growth-filled moments in our lives. Overcoming fear gives us permission to dwell in those moments.

We need to tend to our gardens all through the day. And when we go to sleep, give our thoughts to the Master Gardener, and submit unto the Messiah in all His ways, and the revealing and healing will come. Actively cultivate and plant the good seed with the Master Gardener's direction.

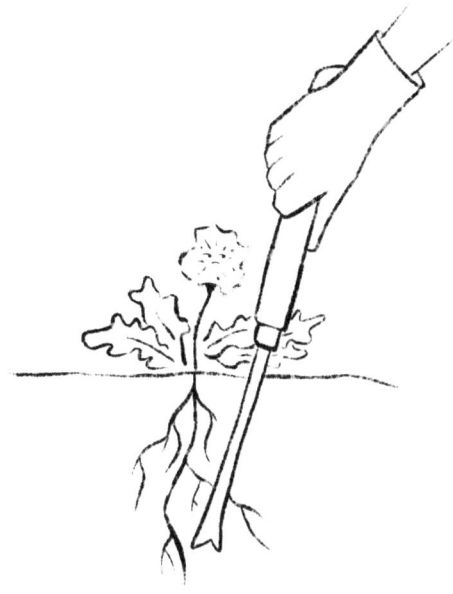

One who tends the fig tree will eat its fruit,
And one who cares for his master will be honored.
As in water a face reflects the face,
So the heart of a person reflects the person.
(Proverbs 27:18–19)

10

Tools from the Master Gardener Study Guide

You came near on the day I called to You;
You said, "Do not fear!"
—Lamentations 3:57

This study is an extra way to enrich and strengthen your research into weeding all areas of your life. I was greatly encouraged as I studied these words and their meanings, and I have confidence that you will also be encouraged.

Words from the garden

The definitions are from Greek and Hebrew/Aramaic words found in *Strong's Exhaustive Concordance of the Bible*.

Garden

Gan *Gan* (Strong's reference H1588): an enclosure, garden.

Paradeisos *Par-ad'-i-sos* (Strong's reference G4237 and G3857): a park, a garden, a paradise.

Tend/Keep/Cultivate/Dress

Abad *Ab-bad'* (Strong's reference H5647 and H5648): to work, serve.

Shamar *Shaw-mar'* (Strong's reference H8104): to keep, watch, preserve.

Ganan *Gaw-nan'* (Strong's reference H1598): gardener, to cover, surround, defend, to hedge about.

Thorn

Akantha *Ak'-an-thah* (Strong's reference G173): a prickly plant, bramble, thorn.

Briar

Batos *Bat'-os* (Strong's reference G942): a bramble bush.

Tare

Zizanion *Dziz-an'-ee-on* (Strong's reference G2215): a kind of darnel or tare resembling wheat, false grain. A fruitless person living without faith from God and therefore is "all show and no go!"

Take root and uproot

Rhizoó *Hrid-zo'-o* (Strong's reference G4492): to cause to take root, plant, fix firmly, establish, to render firm, cause a person or a thing to be thoroughly grounded. Opposite is Ekrizoó: to uproot.

Pheugo *Fyoo'-go* (Strong's reference G1309 and G5437): seeks safety by flight, to escape, to vanish.

Know your enemy: Ephesians 6:12*

Wrestle
Pale *Pal'-ay* (Strong's reference G3823): a contest between two in which each endeavors to throw the other, and which is decided when the victor is able to hold his opponent down with his hand upon his neck.

Principalities
Arche *Ar-khay'* (Strong's reference G746): the person or thing that commences, first person, leader, ruler, etc.

Powers
Exousia *Ex-oo-see'-ah* (Strong's reference G1849): powers of choice, liberty of doing as one pleases, power of authority (influence), of right (privilege), power of rule.

Rulers (of darkness)
Kosmokrator *Kos-mok-fat'-ore* (Strong's reference G2888): lord of the world, prince of this age (Ephesians 2:2).

Spiritual wickedness
Pneumatikos *Pnyoo-mat-ik-os'* (Strong's reference G4152–spiritual): relating to the human spirit, that which possesses the natural soul.

Poneria *Pon-ay-ree'-ah* (Strong's reference G4189–wickedness): depravity, iniquity, malice.

Know what to do: 1 Peter 5:8–9*

Sober
Nepho *Nay'-fo* (Strong's reference G3525): to be calm and collected in spirit, circumspect.

Watchful or Alert
Gregoreuo *Gray-gor-yoo'-o* (Strong's reference G1127): to keep awake, watch, be vigilant.

Steadfast or Establish
Stereos *Ster-eh-os'* (Strong's reference G4731): strong, firm, immovable, solid, stable, sure.

Know your allies: 2 Samuel 22:3*

Trust
Chacah *Khaw-saw'* (Strong's reference H2620): to seek refuge, flee for protection.

Shield
Magen *Maw-gane'* (Strong's reference H4043): to defend, cover, surround.

Salvation
Yesha *Yeh'-shaw* (Strong's reference H3468): deliverance, rescue, safety, welfare, victory.

High tower
Misgab *Mis-gawb'* (Strong's reference H4869): refuge, secure, height, stronghold, inaccessibly high, too high for capture.

Refuge
Manos *Maw-noce'* (Strong's reference H4498): place of escape, to put to flight, to drive hastily, to cause to disappear.

Savior
Yasha *Yaw-shah'* (Strong's reference H3467): be delivered, liberated, saved in battle, to give victory to.

Violence
Chamac *Khaw-mawce'* (Strong's reference H2555): wrong, cruelty, injustice, physical or ethical wrong.

James 5:13–16

Save
Sozo *sode'-zo* (Strong's reference G4982): to save, heal, preserve, rescue.

Raise
Egeiro *eg-i'-ro* (Strong's reference G1453): to waken, rouse (literally from sleep), awake, rise, stand, take up.

The battle is Yahweh's*

Guard
Shamar *Shaw-mar'* (Strong's reference H8104): keep, guard, observe, have charge of, protect, save life.

But if you truly obey his voice and do all that I say, then I will be an enemy to your enemies and an adversary to your adversaries. (Exodus 23:22)

For He will give His angels charge concerning you,
To guard you in all your ways. (Psalm 91:11)

But you will not go out in haste,
Nor will you go as fugitives;
For the Lord will go before you,
And the God of Israel will be your rear guard. (Isaiah 52:12)

. . . who by faith conquered kingdoms, performed acts of righteousness, obtained promises, shut the mouths of lions, quenched the power of fire, escaped the edge of the sword, from weakness were made strong, became mighty in war, put foreign armies to flight. (Hebrews 11:33–34)

Scriptures for the hard days

The following Scriptures are taken from a variety of translations to draw out their meanings. Please take time to look up these verses in your Bible. They will help you and encourage you. They helped and encouraged me in my journey.

Guard your heart above all else, for it determines the course of your life. (Proverbs 4:23)

The steadfast love of the Lord never ceases; his mercies never come to an end; they are new every morning; great is your faithfulness. (Lamentations 3:22–23 English Standard Version)

Do not be conformed to this world, but be transformed by the renewal of your mind, that by testing you may discern what is the will of Yahweh, what is good and acceptable and perfect. (Romans 12:2)

I will give thanks to You, for I am fearfully and wonderfully made;
Wonderful are Your works,
And my soul knows it very well. (Psalm 139:14)

The Lord your God is in your midst,
A victorious warrior.
He will exult over you with joy,
He will be quiet in His love,
He will rejoice over you with shouts of joy. (Zephaniah 3:17)

Delight yourself in the Lord;
And He will give you the desires of your heart. (Psalm 37:4)

Beloved, let us love one another, for love is from God; and everyone who loves is born of God and knows God. (1 John 4:7)

WEEDS

Surely God is good to Israel,
To those who are pure in heart! (Psalm 73:1)

For a righteous man falls seven times, and rises again,
But the wicked stumble in time of calamity. (Proverbs 24:16)

Let all bitterness and wrath and anger and clamor and evil speaking be put away from you, along with all malice. Be kind to one another, tender-hearted, forgiving each other, just as God in Christ also has forgiven you. (Ephesians 4:31–32)

Therefore, having been justified by faith, we have peace with God through our Lord Jesus Christ, through whom also we have obtained our introduction by faith into this grace in which we stand; and we exult in hope of the glory of God. And not only this, but we also exult in our tribulations, knowing that tribulation brings about perseverance; and perseverance, proven character; and proven character, hope; and hope does not disappoint, because the love of God has been poured out within our hearts through the Holy Spirit who was given to us. (Romans 5:1–5)

Make my joy complete by being of the same mind, maintaining the same love, united in spirit, intent on one purpose. (Philippians 2:2)
(The great despair that comes upon the entire world does not have to happen to us. Read all of Philippians 2.)

For God hath not given us the spirit of fear; but of power, and of love, and of a sound mind. (2 Timothy 1:7 KJV)
(Luke 12 is also a good read for this subject.)

Seek ye the Lord while he may be found,
Call ye upon him while he is near:
Let the wicked forsake his way
And the unrighteous man his thoughts;
And let him return unto the Lord,
And He will have mercy upon him,
And to our God,
For He will abundantly pardon.
For My thoughts are not your thoughts,
Nor are your ways My ways, declares the Lord.
For as the heavens are higher than the earth,
So are My ways higher than your ways,
And My thoughts than your thoughts. (Isaiah 55:6–9)

Being born again, not of corruptible seed, but of incorruptible, by the word of God, which liveth and abideth for ever. For all flesh is as grass, and all the glory of man as the flower of grass. The grass withereth, and the flower thereof falleth away: But the word of the Lord endureth for ever. And this is the word which by the gospel is preached unto you. (1 Peter 1:22–25 KJV)

Brethren, if anyone is caught in any trespass, you who are spiritual, restore such a one in a spirit of gentleness; each one looking to yourself, so that you too will not be tempted. (Galatians 6:1–2)

I love the Lord, because he hath heard my voice and my supplications. Because he hath inclined his ear unto me, therefore will I call upon him as long as I live.
(Psalm 116:1–2 KJV)

Who can discern his errors?
Acquit me of hidden faults. (Psalm 19:12)

He who conceals his transgressions will not prosper,
But he who confesses and forsakes them will find
compassion. (Proverbs 28:13)

But if you do not drive out the inhabitants of the land from before you, then it shall come about that those whom you let remain of them will become as pricks in your eyes and as thorns in your sides, and they will trouble you in the land in which you live. (Numbers 33:55)

Scriptures for pruning and weeding

Let me sing now for my well-beloved
A song of my beloved concerning His vineyard.
My well-beloved had a vineyard on a fertile hill.
He dug it all around, removed its stones,
And planted it with the choicest vine.
And He built a tower in the middle of it
And also hewed out a wine vat in it;
Then He expected it to produce good grapes,
But it produced only worthless ones. (Isaiah 5:1–2)

Every branch in Me that does not bear fruit, He takes away; and every branch that bears fruit, He prunes it so that it may bear more fruit. (John 15:2)

Doom to you who call evil good
 and good evil,
Who put darkness in place of light
 and light in place of darkness,
Who substitute bitter for sweet
 and sweet for bitter!

Doom to you who think you're so smart,
 who hold such a high opinion of yourselves!
All you're good at is drinking—champion boozers
 who collect trophies from drinking bouts
And then line your pockets with bribes from the guilty
 while you violate the rights of the innocent.
(Isaiah 5:20–23 The Message)

I will lay it waste;
It will not be pruned or hoed,
But briars and thorns will come up,
I will also charge the clouds to rain no rain on it. (Isaiah 5:6)

Woe to those who call evil good, and good evil;
Who substitute darkness for light and light for darkness;
Who substitute bitter for sweet and sweet for bitter!
(Isaiah 5:20)

And He will judge between the nations, And will render decisions for many peoples; And they will hammer their swords into plowshares and their spears into pruning hooks Nation will not lift up sword against nation, And never again will they learn war. (Isaiah 2:4)

WEEDS

Every branch in Me that does not bear fruit, He takes away; and every branch that bears fruit, He prunes it so that it may bear more fruit. You are already clean because of the word which I have spoken to you. Abide in Me, and I in you. As the branch cannot bear fruit of itself unless it abides in the vine, so neither can you unless you abide in Me. (John 15:2–6)

For those whom the Lord loves He disciplines, and He scourges every son whom He receives. (Hebrews 12:6)

For each tree is known by its own fruit. For men do not gather figs from thorns, nor do they pick grapes from a briar bush. (Luke 6:44)

They speak mere words,
With worthless oaths they make covenants;
And judgment sprouts like poisonous weeds in the furrows of the field. (Hosea 10:4)

But if you do not drive out the inhabitants of the land from before you, then it shall come about that those whom you let remain of them will become as pricks in your eyes and as thorns in your sides, and they will trouble you in the land in which you live. (Numbers 33:55)

For they sow the wind
And they reap the whirlwind.
The standing grain has no heads;
It yields no grain.
Should it yield, strangers would swallow it up. (Hosea 8:7)

But the worthless, every one of them will be thrust away like thorns,
Because they cannot be taken in hand;
But the man who touches them
Must be armed with iron and the shaft of a spear,
And they will be completely burned with fire in their place.
(2 Samuel 23:6–7)

And He spoke many things to them in parables, saying, "Behold, the sower went out to sow; and as he sowed, some seeds fell beside the road, and the birds came and ate them up. Others fell on the rocky places, where they did not have much soil; and immediately they sprang up, because they had no depth of soil. But when the sun had risen, they were scorched; and because they had no root, they withered away. Others fell among the thorns, and the thorns came up and choked them out. And others fell on the good soil and yielded a crop, some a hundredfold, some sixty, and some thirty." (Matthew 13:3–8)

You shall not sow your vineyard with two kinds of seed, or all the produce of the seed which you have sown and the increase of the vineyard will become defiled.
(Deuteronomy 22:9)

Therefore you plant delightful plants
And set them with vine slips of a strange god.
In the day that you plant it you carefully fence it in,
And in the morning you bring your seed to blossom;
But the harvest will be a heap
In a day of sickliness and incurable pain. (Isaiah 17:10–11)

Taken from *The Message*

He told another story. "God's kingdom is like a farmer who planted good seed in his field. That night, while his hired men were asleep, his enemy sowed thistles all through the wheat and slipped away before dawn. When the first green shoots appeared and the grain began to form, the thistles showed up, too.

"The farmhands came to the farmer and said, 'Master, that was clean seed you planted, wasn't it? Where did these thistles come from?'

"He answered, 'Some enemy did this.'

"The farmhands asked, 'Should we weed out the thistles?'

"He said, 'No, if you weed the thistles, you'll pull up the wheat, too. Let them grow together until harvest time. Then I'll instruct the harvesters to pull up the thistles and tie them in bundles for the fire, then gather the wheat and put it in the barn.'"

So he explained. "The farmer who sows the pure seed is the Son of Man. The field is the world, the pure seeds are subjects of the kingdom, the thistles are subjects of the Devil, and the enemy who sows them is the Devil. The harvest is the end of the age, the curtain of history. The harvest hands are angels.

"The picture of thistles pulled up and burned is a scene from the final act. The Son of Man will send his angels, weed out the thistles from his kingdom, pitch them in the trash, and be done with them. They are going to complain to high heaven, but nobody is going to listen. At the same time, ripe, holy lives will mature and adorn the kingdom of their Father." Matthew 13:24–43 (MSG)

* Taken from a Bible study by Hal Geiger, servant minister.

Appendix

Resources for you to explore and enjoy

1. A youth research class created an extensive weed trait list. http://agron-www.agron.iastate.edu/~weeds/Ag317-99/bioeco/weedytraitslist.html

2. Why should you pull those weeds? Question answered from a homestead perspective. https://www.reformationacres.com/2017/06/why-pull-weeds.html

3. I enjoyed this article's perspective of weed pulling as a spiritual art. https://wccm.org/meditators-blog/the-spiritual-art-of-weed-pulling-by-andrew-mcalister/

4. Food allergies, cancer, Lyme disease or any other mycoplasma (bacteria), parasite, or prion blood issue, need a plan to destroy it and heal the body. This is my personal creation from a combination of different plans. http://www.naturalhelpinghands.com/site/2018/01/massive-action/

5. The king of all Lyme, its coinfections, and loads of herbal knowledge https://www.stephenharrodbuhner.com/articles/

6. The full article by Maryn McKenna highlighted in chapter 3 explaining the entire discovery of alpha-gal with some interesting twists and turns. https://mosaicscience.com/story/mammalian-meat-allergy-alpha-gal-allergic-lone-star-tick-bite/

7. A place for those that are mastering their alpha-gal allergy to share their alpha-gal kitchen recipes and experiences without reservations. https://www.facebook.com/groups/TheAlphaGalKitchen/?hc_location=ufi

8. Unlisted food additives can cause major issues. Check out AGI Alpha-gal Information's website. https://alphagalinformation.org/food/

9. A husband and son have alpha-gal and the mother is vegetarian with food allergies https://alphagalcooking.com/our-story/

APPENDIX

10. A place for encouragement for those with alpha-gal, and anything related, such as histamine intolerance and MCAS (mast cell activation syndrome) issues that come along with any allergy/sensitivity. They also have an *Alpha-Gal Content for Select Medications Per Manufacturer,* a list you can ask for that contains safe/unsafe medications, along with many other resources and support. http://www.alphagalencouragers.org/

11. A resource on mammalian meat allergy. https://allergytomeat.wordpress.com/frequently-asked-questions/

12. "The alpha-gal story: Lessons learned from connecting the dots." https://www.jacionline.org/article/S0091-6749(15)00076-7/fulltext

13. Another good resource I found with sound advice: https://www.allergiesalimentairescanada.ca/how-you-can-support-people-with-food-allergies/

14. "My Friend Has a Food Allergy. How Can I Help?" https://kidshealth.org/en/teens/helping-allergies.html

15. This one is, in my opinion, most important in the community. How do restaurants deal with food allergies? https://www.groupon.com/merchant/trends-insights/ trends-by-industry/how-restaurants-can-deal-with-food-allergies

16. Center for Lyme Action is a nonprofit organization dedicated to growing federal funding for Lyme disease to find a cure. https://centerforlymeaction.org/

17. Tick-Borne Conditions United: 2022 LymeTV—Alpha-Gal the "Red Meat Allergy" Panel. https://tbcunited.org/resource/2022-lymetv-alpha-gal-the-red-meat-allergy-panel/

18. Cofounder of Tick-Borne Conditions United, Dr. Jennifer Platt, was appointed to the Department of Health and Human Services' Federal Tick-Borne Disease Working Group (TBDWG). https://tbcunited.org/dr-jennifer-platt-appointed-to-the-federal-tick-borne-disease-working-group/

19. Here's an interesting article from the Springfield News-Leader: https://www.news-leader.com/story/news/local/ozarks/2022/05/08/lone-star-tick-bites-prevalent-missouri-can-cause-alpha-gal-meat-allergy-how-prevent-bites-deet/9679851002/

20. Podcasts, Bible studies, and cooking shows remind you to keep your eyes on Jesus so you can live with more peace and joy. https://faithfulworkouts.com/

Notes

Chapter 1

1. "The Meat Allergy: What It's Like," The Making of Medicine, AVUHealth, March 29, 2018, https://makingofmedicine.virginia.edu/2018/03/29/the-meat-allergy-whats-it-like/

Chapter 3

2. Maryn McKenna, "Why Are So Many People Getting a Meat Allergy?" Mosaic, Wellcome, December 11, 2018, https://mosaicscience.com/story/mammalian-meat-allergy-alpha-gal-allergic-lone-star-tick-bite/

Chapter 7

3. Here is an important article I wrote about the necessity of oxygen in the body. https://www.naturalhelp.net/2021/02/oxygen/

4. Andy Andrews, *The Traveler's Gift: Seven Decisions that Determine Personal Success,* Read by Andy Andrews (Chicago: Oasis Audio, 2012), CD, 4 hr., 53 min.

———. *The Noticer: Sometimes, all a person needs is a little perspective,* Read by Andy Andrews (Nashville: Thomas Nelson, 2009), CD, 4 hr., 9 min.

Brene Brown, *Braving the Wilderness: The Quest for True Belonging and the Courage to Stand Alone,* Read by Brene Brown (New York: Random House Audio, 2017), CD, 4 hr., 12 min.

———. *Daring Greatly: How the Courage to Be Vulnerable Transforms the Way We Live, Love, Parent, and Lead* (New York: Penguin Audio, 2018), CD, 6 hr., 30 min.

Atul Gawande, *Being Mortal: Medicine and What Matters in the End,* Read by Robert Petkoff (New York: Macmillan Audio, 2014), CD, 9 hr., 3 min.

5. Zach Williams, "Fear Is a Liar," track 7 on Chain Breaker, Essential Records, 2016, CD.

Chapter 9

6. Charles Albert Tindley, "Nothing Between," 1905.

About the Author

Jeana Anderson is a therapeutic massage therapist, a national educator of infant massage, a holistic health practitioner, a biofeedback specialist, and a garden enthusiast. Most importantly, she is a daughter of Almighty God, a cherished member of His royal family, given access to the fullness of His love and provision, and co-heir with the Messiah.

She loves being part of a community, teaching, serving others, and learning new things. Growing up on a farm as her parents and grandparents did, and presently living in wooded farmland, she has always taken an interest in health and wellness, natural healing, and simplicity. She has never known any other way of life than an all-natural one.

Jeana is a homemaker and faithful wife who home-schooled her two kids. She is now a working mom with successful adult children. Jeana and her family, who are avid outdoor people, like to travel, hike, kayak, garden, and serve in their church community.

Although she wears many hats, she believes, "These are not what make me what I am; the Almighty Father pours grace upon me to make me what I am. My intentions are to be different, unique, visible, and passionate in what I do, like a magnet that draws because of its characteristics. I ask the Almighty God, my Father, to help me to live today in gratitude, confidence, and purpose."

You can connect with Jeana on her website, Natural Helping Hands (https://naturalhelp.net).

www.ingramcontent.com/pod-product-compliance
Lightning Source LLC
Chambersburg PA
CBHW052032030426
42337CB00027B/4972